THE SONG SPARROW AND THE CHILD

ALSO BY JOSEPH VINING

Legal Identity

The Authoritative and the Authoritarian

From Newton's Sleep

the
SONG SPARROW
and the CHILD

Claims of Science and Humanity

JOSEPH VINING

University of Notre Dame Press
Notre Dame, Indiana

Manufactured in the United States of America

The author and publisher thank Rob Curtis for permission to use
the image of the song sparrow and Graywolf Press, Saint Paul,
Minnesota, and the Estate of Jane Kenyon for permission to
reprint "Who" from Jane Kenyon, *Otherwise: New and Selected
Poems,* copyright 1996 by the Estate of Jane Kenyon.

Library of Congress Cataloging-in-Publication Data
Vining, George Joseph.
The song sparrow and the child : claims of science and humanity /
Joseph Vining.
p.   cm.
Includes bibliographical references (p.   ) and index.
ISBN 0-268-04362-0
I. Science—Moral and ethical aspects.   2. Humanity.
3. Ethics.   I. Title.
BJ57.V56   2004
140—dc22
2003020902

This book is printed on recycled paper.

To Malcolm DeBevoise and George Levine

Contents

Acknowledgments

I wish to acknowledge particular indebtedness to the Rockefeller Foundation Bellagio Center, which nurtured this inquiry; to the Monday Night Group—Huda Akil, neurobiologist, Rudolf Arnheim, psychologist of art, A. L. Becker, linguist, Lee Bollinger, lawyer, John D'Arms, classicist, Kenneth DeWoskin, sinologist, Alice Fulton, poet, Bruce Mannheim, anthropologist, Sabine MacCormack, historian, Piotr Michalowski, linguist, A. K. Ramanujan, poet, James Boyd White, literary critic and lawyer, Christina Whitman, lawyer—with whom the inquiry has been pursued; to the Elkes Fund and the W. W. Cook Trust for the material support each has provided; to Wade McCree, advocate and judge, for the story of "The Pig with a Wooden Leg" in the last chapter; and to readers of the manuscript whose generous criticisms are reflected here—those who read anonymously, together with Charles Eisendrath, journalist, Barbara Hanrahan, publisher, George Levine, literary critic and intellectual historian, John McCausland, priest and lawyer, John Noonan, moral philosopher and judge, Jefferson Powell, theologian and lawyer, Howard Shevrin, experimental psychologist, and Steven Douglas Smith, legal philosopher and lawyer.

THE SONG SPARROW AND THE CHILD

Introduction

TOTALITY AFTER THE TWENTIETH CENTURY

For centuries public claims on behalf of science have been made about our nature and the nature of the world as a whole. Over the twentieth century such claims on behalf of science have grown deeper and stronger. More and more they are total claims, cosmological in the largest sense, and they have evoked opposition equally deep and strong.

There is the scientist in all of us. There is, too, the lawyer and law in all of us, which we realize the moment we serve as a witness or citizen juror. This book explores what the legal mind and ear can contribute to resolving this deep and growing conflict within and among us.

"The question is not whether the theory of the cosmos affects matters, but whether, in the long run, anything else affects them." This was the prescient epigraph William James adopted for his lectures on pragmatism[1] at the beginning of the twentieth century. In it is why this conflict is so deep at the beginning of the twenty-first and its resolution so important for our future together. We know that conventional limits and restraints can change with belief about the ultimate nature of things. The twentieth century has its warning examples, most gruesome where total vision has appeared in social and political thought. The connection between what we think about the nature of the world, and what we allow ourselves to do, is now widely felt, and, with good reason, widely feared.

Our question here will be whether there are, in fact, openings in the total visions of today. The visions are of the facts of the world. What are the facts about the visions? The juror in us might naturally ask of a person testifying to them, "How am I to take what you are saying? Do you actually believe what I hear you to say?" This is empirical inquiry that we all engage in all the time without much thinking how we do it. At our best, especially in important matters, we reach for all the evidence. We listen to all a person says before concluding what any part of it might mean, and we treat what a person does as evidence of the meaning of what a person says.

In this way we will be addressing here how far belief about the ultimate nature of things has actually changed over the twentieth century, in scientist or nonscientist. We will try to let ourselves be told what science is, on behalf of which people speak, and we will wonder how "antiscience" could ever really be a stance to take. Throughout, we will be asking how any total vision of the world can claim the true allegiance of human beings living and thinking together in it.

This book is also about belief—or not—in spirit. The child learns to speak. The song sparrow comes to sing a beautiful song, special not just to its kind but to its individual throat and tongue. They are often compared, the development of individual song in the song sparrow and language in the child. Experiments that would be gruesome and called atrocity in a human context are performed on the young song sparrow. What is it that holds us back from performing the same experiment on the child—or letting it be done? What really, in thought and actual belief today?

On such large questions touching our basic view of each other and ourselves, and other creatures too such as the song sparrow, we should be having a conversation or open meditation. The discussion ought not to be primarily argumentative, as we tend to understand argument. Binding you to me by successful moves of my mind would lose all that can be hoped for. It cannot be merely descriptive, with us absent from the picture. Nor should it try to move from one proposition to another whose meaning or truth depends on having done with the first. In any conversation or meditation we return more than once to the questions and examples with which we begin, and we will do so here. An earlier book of mine took a form that was meant to merge with and give the reader an experience of its subject, which was the legal form of thought. The form of this book too reflects what we are talking about, a world that really does include ourselves.

Chapter One

THE SONG SPARROW
AND THE CHILD

TRUTH AND ACTION

None of us can escape the connection between a larger sense of things—a sense of the nature of the world—and what we ourselves do and what our contribution is to the way the world will be. Politics and ethics, and what we say is atrocity after it has happened, are never far from the steps we take toward or away from a cosmology. Consider these twentieth-century accounts of the nature of things and how we learn about the nature of things. Put together with them these other accounts of what human beings have done to one another over this same century, in the second column. Then let us ask the questions that together they raise.

The song sparrow and the child side by side in the first passage are not too small a pair to begin with. Young song sparrows are deafened in experiments on them. Why not experimentally deafen a child? It is in us to do it, or let it be done. The child's own hands are too weak to protect his ears. What in thought and actual belief stands between us and deafening a child as we might deafen a sparrow?

"A song sparrow sings his elaborate song, stereo-typed in its general message but ornamented by himself alone. . . . If deafened as a nestling, he will sing nothing beyond a kind of buzz. . . .

"Childhood is the time for language, no doubt about it. Young children, the younger the better, are good at it; it is child's play. . . . I possessed a splendid collection of neurons nested in a center . . . probably similar to the center in a songbird's brain . . . used for learning the species' song while still a nestling. Like mine, the bird's center is only there for studying in childhood; if he hears the proper song at that stage he will have it in mind for life, ornamenting it later with brief arpeggios so that it becomes his own, particular, self-specific song. . . . But if he cannot hear it as a young child, the center cannot compose it on its own, and what comes out later when he is ready for singing and mating is an unmelodious buzzing noise. This is one of the saddest tales in experimental biology." (Lewis Thomas, *The Fragile Species*, 1992)[1]

Would it be a sadder tale if such things were done also to a child?

"Unit 731 proved scientifically . . . the best treatment for frostbite. . . . [T]hose seized for medical experiments . . . were taken outside in freezing weather and left with exposed arms, periodically drenched with water, until a guard decided that frostbite had set in. . . . [T]his was determined after the 'frozen arms, when struck with a short stick, emitted a sound resembling that which a board gives when it is struck. . . .'

"Unit 731 . . . experimented on a three-day-old baby, measuring the temperature with a needle stuck inside the infant's middle finger. 'Usually a hand of a three-day-old infant is clenched into a fist . . . but by sticking the needle in, the middle finger could be kept straight to make the experiment easier.'" (*New York Times Report on Human Experimentation in Manchuria, 1932–1945,* 1995)[2]

"Since there was a marked difference in our animal research on epilepsy between the behavior of older and younger specimens, we tested epileptic children under similar conditions in pressure chambers. Up until now only children between 11 and 13 were at our disposal. At a pressure corresponding to 4 to 6,000 meters no epileptic attacks occurred. In humans age 11 to 13 corresponds to 5 to 6 months of age in rabbits, an age at which the cramp threshold, as is also the case with rabbits, is not so low as to induce cramps with certain regularity under pressure chamber conditions. To have a basis of comparison, we would need to test epileptic children between 5 and 6 years of age." (1943 grant application to the German Research Foundation by Hans Nachtsheim, later and postwar of the Max Planck Institute of Comparative Genetic Biology and Genetic Pathology, and the Hans Nachtsheim Prize for Theoretical Research in Human Genetics. Christian Pross and Götz Aly, *The Value of the Human Being: Medicine in Germany 1918–1945,* 1991)[3]

Where is the line between the animal and the child?

"Basic to our world view is the idea that human beings and other higher animals are part of the biological order like any other organisms. . . . [T]he biologically specific characteristics of these animals—such as their possession of a rich system of consciousness . . . their capacity for language . . . their capacity for rational thought . . . —are biological phenomena like any other biological phenomena. . . . [L]ike it or not, it is the world view we have. Given what we know about the details of the world . . . this world view is not an option. It is not simply up for grabs along with a lot of competing world views. . . .

"We live in exactly one world, not two or three or seventeen . . . a world that consists entirely of physical particles in fields of force, and in which some of these particles are organized into systems that are conscious biological beasts, such as ourselves. . . .

"It would be tricky to try to define the notion of a system, but the simple intuitive idea is that systems are collections of particles where the spatio-temporal boundaries of the system are set by causal relations. . . . Babies, elephants, and mountain ranges are . . . examples of systems." (John Searle, *The Rediscovery of the Mind*, 1992; *The Construction of Social Reality*, 1995)[4]

Where is the line between the animate and the inanimate?

"I am inclined to accept . . . that living creatures just are very complicated physico-chemical mechanisms." (J. J. C. Smart, philosopher of science, in *Minds and Machines: Contemporary Perspectives in Philosophy Series*, ed. Alan Ross Anderson, 1964)[5]

"Any definition of complexity is necessarily context-dependent, even subjective. . . . In actuality, then, we are discussing one or more definitions of complexity that depend on a description of one system by another system, presumably a complex adaptive system, which could be a human observer." (Murray Gell-Mann, Nobel Prize in Physics, *The Quark and the Jaguar: Adventures in the Simple and the Complex*, 1994)[6]

"An organism is merely a transition, a stage between what was and what will be. Reproduction represents both the beginning and the end, the cause and the aim. . . . Every object that biology studies is a system of systems. Being part of a higher-order system itself, it sometimes obeys rules that cannot be deduced simply by analysing it. . . .

"What could impose a limit on understanding the living world was . . . no longer a difference in nature between the living and the inanimate worlds. It was the inadequacy of our means. . . . Biologists no longer study life today. They no longer attempt to define it. Instead, they investigate the structure of living systems, their functions, their history. . . .

"The qualities, functions and development of a living organism thus simply express the interactions between its components. Underlying each character are the properties of certain structures. . . . [I]ntellectual performance as observed in an individual . . . reflects . . . structures hidden in the depth of the brain, which function at many levels of integration, but to which there is presently no experimental access. . . .

"Biology has demonstrated that there is no metaphysical entity hidden behind the word 'life.' . . . From particles to man, there is a whole series of integration, of levels, of discontinuities. But there is no breach either in the composition of the objects or in the reactions that take place in them; no change in 'essence.'" (François Jacob, Nobel Prize in Medicine and Physiology, *The Logic of Life: A History of Heredity*, 1982; *The Possible and the Actual*, 1982)[7]

"Large objects wrapped in straw were passed from the train to the Ping Fan technicians. . . . [T]wo live humans were inside each bag. The bags were so tightly bound that the prisoners head and feet touched each other. . . . Laboratory technicians would then go to either building 7 or 8, order guards to provide the number of 'logs' needed for the next experiment, and prepare the laboratory to receive victims." (Sheldon H. Harris, *Factories of Death,* 1994)[8]

"Knowing what we do about a 'total institution' like S-21, . . . how can we explain what happened there? . . . [Studies of the Nazi camps] illuminate the culture of obedience that suffuses total institutions and the numbing dehumanization that occurs, among perpetrators and victims alike. . . . Studies of the Holocaust also bring us face to face with the indifference that the Nazis, like the Cambodians, showed their victims. . . . [T]he people working in the Nazi camps and at S-21 were not inherently brutal or authoritarian. . . . [T]he workers at S-21, like the prisoners, were trapped inside a merciless place and a pitiless scenario. . . .

"The Party Center adopted the doctrine that the leaders of a Communist Party . . . were empowered . . . because of their privileged relationship to historical laws. . . . Turning the victims into 'others,' in a racist fashion—and using words associated with animals to describe them—made them easier to mistreat and easier to kill. . . .

"S-21 . . . was a Cambodian, Communist, imported, twentieth-century phenomenon. . . . [B]ut the perpetrators' indifference to the pain of others retains a capacity to shock. We wait in vain for hints that what the workers did damaged their relations with each other, jarred their calligraphy, or disturbed their sleep. . . . [It] was no more complicated or distressing, it seems, than hosing down a pavement or plowing up a field." (David Chandler, *Voices from S-21: Terror and History in Pol Pot's Se-cret Prison*, 1999)⁹

And so we could go on, glancing now at examples of twentieth-century thought about the place and nature of the human in the cosmos, now at twentieth-century action that tugs upon the sleeve and asks what connections there are, what lines there are:

"I grant that the brain is a tool of investigation, that it has nothing of the divine about it, that it owes nothing to any transcendence whatsoever. . . . To affirm the exis-tence of a mathematical reality independent of percep-tion certainly doesn't amount to making a teleological claim. . . . No mathematician would make such an argu-ment! In no way, then, can my position be characterized as teleological. . . ." (Alain Connes, Fields Medalist, in *Conversations on Mind, Matter and Mathematics*, 1995)[10]

"The more the universe seems comprehensible, the more it also seems pointless." (Steven Weinberg, Nobel Prize in Physics, *The First Three Minutes: A Modern View of the Origin of the Universe*, 1977)[11]

"Why should it have a point? . . . It's just a physical system, what point is there? I've always been puzzled by that statement." (Margaret Geller, astronomer, quoted in Steven Weinberg, *Dreams of a Final Theory*, 1992)[12]

"There may well be only one, or a small number, of complete unified theories . . . that are self-consistent and allow the existence of structures as complicated as human beings. . . . [I]f we do discover a complete theory, it should in time be understandable in broad principle by everyone, not just a few scientists." (Stephen W. Hawking, *A Brief History of Time,* 1988)[13]

QUESTIONS FOR OUR FUTURE

Suppose a vision of the universe is true in which system and process have a total reach. Can there ultimately be a difference between the way a human being is treated in the pursuit of knowledge by experimental method, and the way an animal is now treated?

Ultimately there will be no difference in treatment if any such total theory of the universe, theory of everything including ourselves, is true.

Is there any connection between the *total* in twentieth-century totalitarian social and political thought, and the *total* in visions today that exhaust the nature of the world—the cosmologies now urged so strongly, the final theories that are now sought?

There is a connection. It lies in the connection between human thought and human action and is traced in the line, protecting us from one another, that our action does or does not cross in pursuit of experimental method or in daily life.

Do those among us who teach and urge the total visions now become familiar, visions of the world as a world only of system and process, believe them to be true?

I do not think they believe what they seem to say. The scientist or mathematician speaking cosmologically does not cease to be a human person speaking, and acting.

Need there be science? Yes. There is something of a necessity to science, like the necessity of eating or sleeping, like the necessity of trusting.

Need there be antiscience, enemies of science? No. There need be no such deep and unbridgeable gulf among us or within us.

But the totalitarian experienced in modern history lends urgency to the inquiry into totality we enter here. In our inquiry we will press toward human candor, simple in its way, simply candor with ourselves as with others. Human candor alone, among us and within us, may be a wonderfully large part of what we want if we are all to acknowledge the deep necessity of science, the scientist in each of us, and use the power gained by the scientific enterprise without self-destruction.

Why *human* candor? What other sort of candor is there? Remember the milk of *human* kindness. For some there is kindness in animals, for some there is divine kindness or nature is kind. So with candor. Our own is our responsibility; we should not rule out at the beginning a capacity for it elsewhere.

Total Theory

If questions of this kind have intrigued or haunted you as they have intrigued and haunted me, and if the inclination of answers such as these might be your own, then working with these pages may be helpful.

The fear engendered by late-twentieth-century discussions of the nature of the world is in part fear of ourselves, underlined by what the experience of this same century has taught us gifted and ordinary alike about our capabilities, especially what we are capable of doing and watching done to our fellow human beings.

But fear and hostility today are also in part a result of our reading and understanding language, human language, as total visions of the world would invite us to do. Human language has been presented to us, in schools and beyond, to be read as if we and it were in a world in which there were no persons speaking. What is said has been not read as a whole but abstracted into proposition or formula, to be argued over, defended with scorn, or attacked with fear.

Just as it is true there is the scientist in each of us, it is also true we each speak a human language, scientist as well as nonscientist. We need not forget, indeed we must not forget that valuable as proposition and formula are, human language is not ultimately read confined in this way. Again, the scientist or mathematician speaking cosmologically does not cease to be a human person speaking and acting.

Our concern here will be with visions that are presented as visions of everything, cosmologies called "theory" partly because of the widespread association of the word "theory" with an interest in system and process. They are distinct from the general thought or vision we routinely call "comprehensive," that seeks to be as consistent as it can and keeps to the hope of coherence. Total theories are marked by their exclusiveness. In them the world, the universe, the cosmos, is introduced with the excluding phrases "nothing but" or "nothing more than," "only," "merely," followed by the details of the total vision being urged.

To focus upon total theories in their particulars, I have chosen several books of the latter part of the twentieth century which I think will be representative, and the quality of which will not be seriously disputed. These are Lewis Thomas's *The Fragile Species,* the last of his wonderful series that began with *The Lives of a Cell;* the Nobelist François Jacob's *The Logic of Life* and *The Possible and the Actual;* the Nobelist Jacques Monod's *Chance and Necessity;* the Nobelist Steven Weinberg's *Dreams of a Final Theory;* and the *Conversations on Mind, Matter and Mathematics* of the well-known neurobiologist Jean-Pierre Changeux and the mathematician and Fields Medalist Alain Connes. I have kept this book short and hope that my references to these examples will be sufficient. The reader may want to have the selection at hand, where they can speak for themselves.

Many other examples of total theory could be picked out. I have included an expanded selection in a list of further readings at the end. One of the most powerful, and not by a working scientist or mathematician, is Elias Canetti's *Crowds and Power,* a total theory of the human evoked by the agony of twentieth-century totalitarianism. I have had at my side others' efforts to approach some of the problems with which we will be concerned here. Among them are the computer scientist Joseph Weizenbaum's *Computer Power and Human Reason,* the philosopher John Searle's *The Rediscovery of the Mind* and *The Construction of Social Reality,* the cultural historian Jacques Barzun's *Darwin, Marx, Wagner,* the cosmological physicist

Roger Penrose's *The Emperor's New Mind* and *Shadows of the Mind*, the physicist Freeman Dyson's *Infinite in All Directions, Disturbing the Universe,* and *Imagined Worlds,* and the clinical neurologist Oliver Sacks's *Awakenings* and *The Man Who Mistook His Wife for a Hat.* I have included in the further readings these and other works that have wrestled from the mid-twentieth century on with the problems we now face, including works by the chemist and philosopher of science Michael Polanyi, who so felt the pressure of the totalitarian upon cosmological thought.

TOTAL THEORY AND THE READER'S OWN DECISION

Recall the daily common mystery, that each of us is alone and not alone, here and not just here, now and not only now. This we learn in life. It is not often heard in school or college, simply because of the grip which the kind of thought necessary to the operation of machines tends to have on thought itself today.

Social and economic machines, pieces of engineering technology, the bodily machine in medicine: they all operate and are thought about in daily life on an assumption of either-or, that something is one thing or another thing, but not both at the same time. This is the very basis of the computer, the switch that can be on or off, the gate in the transistor that is open or closed. It is enshrined in number, where 1 is not 2. In the view of life permitted by this kind of thought, "switching off" is the image of death.

This part of thought necessary to the design and operation of machines is important enough, and it should be enough, for those working with this part of thought, that it is so important. But time and again it is presented as thought itself, all there is at least for us at the human level of the world we inhabit. Thought based on these assumptions is not all there is. I do not mean merely that there is also a domain of quantum mechanics in physics. Thought based on these assumptions is not the way you can think about human beings, and continue to do the thinking—even the kind of thinking involved in the design or maintenance of social or technological or bodily machines. What enables you to continue, and thought itself therefore to continue, is perception of another reality and of a necessity that is as true and necessary as gravity is true and necessary.

The way you think about human beings and yourself, which underlies and supports human law also, has no place in it for categorical distinctions between what you create and what is given to you, or between what is now, what was then, and what is to come, no place in it for these distinctions and axioms of thought so useful in so many subjects but worse than useless in thinking about yourself. These are the same distinctions and axioms that make it possible to conceive of putting some words together and saying something along the lines of the advertisement on the planetarium billboard, "Come Visit Our Planetarium, You Tiny Insignificant Speck in the Universe." For a planetarium seeking paying customers this is a joke of course, obviously meant as a joke; there would be no joke in it, if there were not a way of thought beyond.

Much of the argument over total theory, we will find, is argument about human significance in the vastness of the cosmos as we have become able to see it in the course of the twentieth century. If you, the reader, come to the point where you think you cannot see anything beyond what would make you a "tiny, insignificant speck in the universe," give yourself the respect of reading yourself closely and as a whole. Do what lawyers do with witnesses' testimony, but more politely since you will be the witness. We may think we believe something here, or do not believe something there, but we do not have the last word on what we believe unless we read ourselves as a whole, in the same way we read others to determine what it is they are really saying and what it is they actually believe.

It is a task, work, to read ourselves, just as it is work really to read another. There is nothing automatic about it, nothing formulaic about it. You do me the honor to work at reading me—as if what I really believed mattered to you; were I watching I might be brought to conclude, whatever I may think of my worth, that there is no mere "as if" in your attention. You do the same honor to yourself, grant respect to yourself, in working to read yourself as if it mattered—to yourself—what you really believe and think. You grant to yourself authority in that way, as you grant authority to another in that way.

Read others. The strictest "rationalist," most fastidious in his arguments, who has a dog, who nuzzles it and cares for it, and weeps when it dies, may not be a strict rationalist in actual belief. Read yourself, paying attention to what you say and do, giving it the same close reading as a whole that you were taught to give to the various authorities presented to you, or that you give them now. Then, for yourself, you too will be an authority, ultimately the final authority on the largest questions of all.

FACT AND THE PERSON

But let me make something of a lawyer's apology, especially since we will be referring in a later chapter to the mathematician G. H. Hardy's lovely little book *A Mathematician's Apology.*

Everyone moving to a position on what he or she believes is in something of the position of a lawyer. Everyone is attending to testimony: to her own testimony to herself, constant if very lucky, various, more likely, at different times and in different contexts; and to the testimony of others, apparently quite various, in substance and in language both, with words and constructions of words variously nuanced even within the same family growing up together, and shading more quickly than we like into the immediately perceptible objective differences that present the task of translating.

A lawyer has no authority to state any conclusion about which mathematicians spend their lives debating, or scientists of various training, or medical doctors of whom Lewis Thomas is so fine an example. Lawyers have no authority, that is, in the sense that the lawyer's statement or conclusion is one that need be paid any attention by scientists or doctors once they have done with lawyers.

But to the lawyer, as to the citizen who acts as juror and participates in the legal form of thought and in decision about action and restraint of action, doctors or scientists or mathematicians are witnesses. Their expertise and claim to be listened to as experts having been established on what is called *voir dire,* they appear on both sides of an issue. Efforts are made to avoid having to face and evaluate dissent among those whose authority is based upon a conclusion that their reasoning, and the language in which they couch it, cannot be fully followed without an education too long for lawyer or juror to undertake—and, perhaps, a gift as well. But the lawyer knows that what appears in thought, speech, and analysis as a "fact" and what is referred to as a "fact" in contrast to some other element of thought, speech, or analysis, remains a fact only until it is challenged. Then it is a decision, and however strenuously it may be called a fact, after the fact as it were, it is still a decision, a decision "of fact," as lawyers say, which accompanies (and is entwined with) decisions "of law." The decision-maker believes there is fact, such a thing as fact, and that the outcome of the decision is such; but the decision, made necessary by the challenge, never disappears, nor the person who makes the decision.

APPEAL

From the outside, the presence of dissent on a vision of the world, within mathematics, or science, or a particular field of either, puts each who proposes a vision of the world into the position of making an appeal. Appeal they do. They do not ignore. Aggression and ridicule are a turn to and a focus upon the outside, from what is assumed to be the inside, as suspicion and scolding (and, indeed, shunning and ignoring and exclusion) work to bring about the appearance of greater assent within. What is the "scientific view"? What does "mathematics" tell us? If there is one challenge, one dissent by a scientist or mathematician to what another says *is* the view of science or what mathematics tells us, there is an inescapable judgment to be made by the nonscientist and the nonmathematician.

Our inclination might be to say this cannot be so, that the matter should or even must be left to scientists or mathematicians themselves; and those within the disciplines, making their appeals, will urge this also. Certainly there are elements of the human phenomenon of authority within what the mathematician Alain Connes terms "the small community of mathematicians," and also within the larger community of "scientists." Deference, central texts, presupposition of good faith and more are there to be seen. But there is in fact no authority within these communities to determine the view of science or the nature of mathematics for those outside.

Each scientist and mathematician determines for himself these questions even if he does not distinguish between his own view and the view of that which is beyond himself and with which he identifies. Since it cannot be resolved in any sufficiently conclusive way who is and who is not within these communities, the possibility of looking for some core of agreement within them by filtering out the differences of each member and looking at the residue is not available, even if their language were so common and so neatly contained in boxes that it could be manipulated to such a conclusion; and, in any event, a single challenge would push the decision back to the observer and listener outside.

But there should be no battle lines drawn and confrontation across them. Where a vision of *all* the world is presented, it extends to us, and to our language, and to our own experience, which we outside use and on which we have our own beliefs and views. That should not be forgotten. We will turn to it whenever we touch upon the hope for us all that lies in human candor. On the matter of language alone, we are in a situation where there is never authority to legislate the use and meaning of words or expressions or even linguistic structures and constructions (what is often termed "syntax" as opposed to "semantics"). Statistics of use, numbers, are pointers only.

Here, in this inquiry into total vision absorbing language and all else, we meet the substantive rather than linguistic consequences of our situation. Or instead of substantive consequences we may say the consequences for belief. They flow from the fact, associated with what we will call in later chapters the necessity of assent, that we are split, that there are more than one of us. All of us face this as a fact of the world, curious and puzzling though it is, as curious and puzzling as the "unreasonable effectiveness of mathematics"[14] in the world. If we do not accept it we are treated as mad and then meet a force, another fact, the force and fact, yes, of law.

Human, yet split. We can stand back and ask—is the human being capable of love? If we think the majority of living human beings do not love, what do we conclude about human capacity? If, following Abraham's plea with God before the destruction of the cities of the plain, we conclude that not just the majority but the vast majority of living human beings do not love, what do we conclude then about human capacity? The inner sense of humanity is not known by numbers, however great the majority. What do we conclude if there is only one human being who loves in all the world? Identity is strained—but if it holds?

The situation, our situation, is not different when total theories of the world are presented. Whether the theory is singular in its totalism and dissent is to its totalism, or the theory is one of various contending total theories, there is a judgment to be made about ourselves, about the theorist, and about the theory. So, we begin with an appeal by one who wishes to prevail. But where the appeal is in favor of a total theory, the appeal is to something beyond the theory. That something, call it the person who is judging and making the decision, is then introduced into the situation, as is the appeal and the person making the appeal. The person making the appeal is as it were *looking at* the person who will judge and decide, looking at *her* or *him.* Or we may come back to you, the reader—the person making the appeal may be appealing to you directly. There is *seeing,* on the one side; *him* or *her,* or *you,* on the other. The theory's closedness is broken open, to the person beyond. And though you accept a theory and its totality, as explaining your acceptance and the language you understand and the theorizing of the theorist, there is still a judgment being made, and you the person judging are still there, as the him or her whom you observe from afar facing an appeal in school or in life, and accepting it, is still there. The theory is not all there is before you, as all the world is all there is before you, strange and puzzling though some of it or all of it may be.

Acceptance of a total theory, assent to it, could be a form of death, a giving up, a farewell. I suppose we can truly assent to death, truly accept it when it comes by our own hand as well as when it comes by forces beyond our control. Though work with suicides suggests a sense in which we are "not ourselves" when we seek our own death, certainly it seems we can assent to death identifying with another who will live, for the sake of an individual or the world. How much further we can go without such identification no one knows.

But in accepting total theory, the giving up is a choice: at the moment of acceptance, when accepted, the theory is not total.

And after acceptance? Is this *giving,* which is beyond the theory, this giving over of oneself, this holding out of one's hands, a giving up to sleep rather than death? Is there no return? Is there no memory of the judgment made, and does what fills the mind after acceptance not include that opening in it out to the person to whom the appeal was made and, through the person, beyond? Once a person is actually acknowledged—when a person is seen, which we cannot do all the time and get on with life but sometimes it happens to us that we do—it is a moment of the marvelous, a marvel. You fall back, your mind is filled as if by music. Think of the representation of "thought" that is so often met in total theories, whether that of the realist mathematician, or that of the geneticist or neurobiologist or cognitive scientist: thought itself is a representation or a mirroring, a doubling of something in the outside world. If thought is representation, what would the representation be of, if what is reflected within were a person, one of us?

Chapter Two

THE CLOSE READING
OF COSMOLOGIES

The late Lewis Thomas sang to me, perhaps to you, certainly to many. He sang of the wonders of the living world, the fascination, charm, curiosity, and surprise of it. *The Lives of a Cell,*[1] *The Medusa and the Snail,*[2] and the other collections of his essays were in a form and style, personal, allusive, short, that he made very much his own. He was open to music, sensitive to it, moved by it; he wrote of music—*Late Night Thoughts on Listening to Mahler's Ninth Symphony.*[3] He tried his own hand at poetry—poetry for him was not something others with looser minds might do. He administered great medical institutions. He was a wonderful man and I keep his books on a special shelf.

Lewis Thomas was also a timid man. Wonderful, inspiring, good to read and be with, but oppressed, and ultimately timid. It is this oppression and timidity with which we should begin, and see in Thomas precisely because he is an exemplary figure. Then we will move in later chapters to other figures to pull out the source of Thomas's timidity and the source of a problem all educated people know today and which the so-called uneducated sense. It is not merely a problem. It is also a fear, after the twentieth century and its demonstration of what human beings can do to one another.

We can then look, in our discussion here, and beyond it, to those figures in science who have themselves addressed the problem and the fear. Joseph Weizenbaum, the distinguished computer scientist and pioneer in computer programming, is one who we can imagine taking Thomas's hand, and to whom Thomas might listen as seriously as to those he feels looking over his shoulder. Weizenbaum has voiced the connection there may possibly be, between what the educated are now willing to say in learned journals and in classrooms, and a doing of what we have seen human beings do to one another in the twentieth century. He may stand at the end as an example of why we can have hope and even confidence that we moved into a better and not a worse time with the change in the first digit in our yearly accounts.

SCIENCE AND ANTISCIENCE

Lewis Thomas's last book, *The Fragile Species*,[4] is an account of cooperation, symbiosis, and mutual dependence. In its most general aspect it is an essay on the problem of units of reference, what is to be viewed as separate and what not, or, in aesthetic and perceptual terms, what is a detail of a whole and, if so, of what whole it is a detail. Ultimately it is an appeal that the earth itself be seen as an organism of which man is a part much as an organelle is a part of a cell, drawing from it but dependent on it also.

But toward the end of *The Fragile Species* Thomas darkens. "Science itself could be going out of favor in the public mind." He senses and laments a "new atmosphere of anti-science, more than a fear of science . . . , sweeping through the most educated and well-informed segments of the population. . . . [W]e might as well recognize that anti-science is reaching the status of a philosophical position in the public mind, and we had better face up to it." (pp. 189–90)

What, in Thomas's view, is "science," opposed to which is this "antiscience"? Read to the very end of the book, and part of the answer appears: what "science" might be deemed to be by those who are admitted to the company of scientists, and why there might be "antiscience"—what Jacques Monod writing twenty years earlier also

saw as "the fear if not the hatred—in any case the estrangement—
felt toward scientific culture by so many people today."⁵

Thomas speaks in his concluding chapter of the possibility that
beyond human minds the earth itself, as a living organism, has a
mind. But he ends, this his last book, with an apology. "My scientist
friends will not be liking this notion. . . . [M]y friends will object to
the word 'mind,' worrying that I am proposing something mystical, a
governor of the earth's affairs, a Presence, something *in charge*. . . ."
(p. 192)

Earlier he had noted the "antipathy within the biological community, especially among evolutionary biologists" to the proposal
called the "Gaia Hypothesis" that "life on the planet has been chiefly
responsible for the regulation of that life's own environment." "They
do not much like the name, for one thing, with its undertones of
deity and deification. . . . [T]hey object to the idea that evolution can
plan ahead for future contingencies." (pp. 119–20) Each time Thomas
recalls such dislike and objection he responds by reciting a belief, as
if with obedience but, being the man he is, indicating his discomfort.
Here at this earlier point before he ends, his recitation is an emphasis with italics that when life appears, "a *system*" comes "into existence," which if "sufficiently complex . . . automatically provides a
series of choices among strategies for future contingencies." In the
context of acknowledged antipathy around him, he confesses that
when the contingencies appear "it has the look of planning and purposiveness." Not purposiveness, only the look of purposiveness.

Then at the end (pp. 192–93), responding to the dislike of his
"scientist friends" and their worry about mysticism and presence, he
says, "Not a bit of it, or maybe only a little bit; my fantasy is of a different nature." Not a bit of it, or maybe "only a little bit." He goes on
to explain that the greater mind he wonders about is "merely there,"
an important part of the belief he confesses. The terms "merely" and
"only" and "no more than" sound again and again. "It is merely there,
an immense collective thought, spread everywhere, unconcerned
with the details."

And "unconcern with the details" is also important, because any
individual molecule, individual sparrow, individual child, is unim-
portant, replaceable, passing, merely part of a process. There is no

real place for the concrete, the particular, not to speak of a particular such as one human being that has a transcendent value.

"It is, if it exists," he continues in his apology for wondering about a greater mind, "the *result* of the earth's life, not at all the cause." He recites the total vision underlying what today are called "emergent properties," that all, all, everything, everything, is ultimately and no more than a "property"—the term being taken over from human law, where we all use it, and from mathematics and the description of mathematical objects. Everything is a property of a thing, that can be grasped. If it is not initially given, it "emerges" as systems are combined with systems. The *result,* not at all the cause.

"What does it do, this mind of my imagining, if it does not operate the machine? It contemplates, that's what it does, is my answer. No big deal, I tell my scientist friends; not to worry."

Here is the source of antiscience, if this is science. "This" if this be science includes both the content of a creed, and the particular character and attitude exposed in pressing it. No speaker of a creed, not even the speaker of a creed meant to be universal, can avoid infusing into it his own reasons for speaking it. If the speaker has no reasons, then the words spoken begin to take on the quality of noise, branches rubbing together in the wind. Here "science," as it appears in Thomas's words, is both a denial of purpose or presence, anything that is beyond process and result, both this and, as well, "antipathy" to or "dislike" of purpose or of presence, or of belief in purpose and presence, or of utterance of purpose and presence.

There is a denial that we exist who are present to one another, who seek and care and have concern, and speak of care and concern, who are identified indeed with our purpose and our care, and who care for the particular and the concrete: a denial that we exist, and at the same time a hostility to the utterance and the belief uttered that we do exist.

Jews in Germany knew something of the feeling of being the target of an attitude of this kind, a denial that they were human, subhuman they were called, animals, and a hostility toward them too, vermin they were called, a hostility so suspicious, so strong, that it could well be taken as driving the affirmative part of the thought of those expressing such an attitude. Blacks made "properties" in slavery and blacks after slavery have known something of the same, a denial that they were human, accompanied by a dislike of their skin. It takes the strongest character, perhaps indeed one religiously based in the synagogue or the black church, to forgive such an attitude and not become similarly "anti-" in response.

The denial and the hostility here are different though. All humanity is the target. Those expressing such an attitude are themselves included. And that being the case, the response here where all are included can be not just searching for an "explanation" of the hostility—which might adopt much of the total vision of the attacker—but rather, and as well, an inquiry into actual belief, asking for candor, which asking can be done without hostility because in itself it is according a dignity to the one of whom the demand is made.

"Science" to which Thomas speaks at the end of his work need not be this way. *The Fragile Species* itself is an appeal for public support of science and a paean to the excitement and wonder that a true openness to the natural world—and, in Thomas's case as in so many others, what can only be called a love of the natural world—can bring to one's own life on earth. There are great scientists from Newton to Einstein who are not troubled by divinity, nor driven by a desire to eliminate it from the thought and speech of all. Some skilled and inspired practitioners of science have difficulty with the divine, some do not. It would be difficult to achieve any consensus on whether there is a connection between greatness in science and difficulty or absence of difficulty with the divine. After all, Moses said, "Why me?" and "Let me see your face," and the apostle Thomas was Doubting Thomas. Darwin doubted his own capacity to encompass the whole, lamenting at the end of his life the stunting of his aesthetic sense.

Scientific method is a gift, to particular men and women and through them to mankind, as music is a gift to particular men and women and to mankind. Nature has been responsive, good to us as we have pursued this method of inquiry. Mathematics accompanying science has made possible much of its achievement, and mathematical insight is an illumination, a gift to men and women "gifted," as we say, with mathematical capacities. There is no intrinsic incompatibility between the perception and creation of systems or finding beauty in them, and acknowledging there is in the world of our experience that which is beyond system.

Animus, "dislike," "antipathy" and its ugliness, would seem indeed much more a feature of the late twentieth century than of the history of science as such. It is, certainly, the language of war that one meets at the end of the Nobelist Steven Weinberg's *Dreams of a Final Theory,*[6] which is contemporaneous with Thomas's *Fragile Species.* After remarking how the "process of demystification has accelerated in this century" (p. 246), he recounts his participation in the debate over what is to be taught young children: "My answer did not satisfy the senator because he knew as I did what would be the effect of a course in biology that gives an appropriate emphasis to the theory of evolution. As I left the committee room, he muttered that 'God is still in heaven anyway.' Maybe so, but we won that battle; Texas high-school textbooks are now not only allowed but required to teach the modern theory of evolution, and with no nonsense about creationism. But there are many places (today especially in Islamic countries) where this battle is yet to be won and no assurance anywhere that it will stay won." (p. 249)

Strange, this struggle over the minds of young children—one might think that the theory of evolution, appealing, simple, fertile, fascinating, like a beautiful equation in mathematics, could fend for itself when presented to curious young minds. But beyond it, the battle to which Weinberg refers extends to uses of force in the systems of adult society, with jealous monitoring of who is to be included and who excluded from the community that speaks for science.

Much of the evidence for any impression about the atmosphere of our own time is in what the offeror of it has been led to read by chance and instinct. One can only ask whether one's impression is similar to others' impressions that are similarly based on what they have heard and been led to read by chance and instinct. No statistical poll can be taken, when the question at issue is who qualifies to be polled, no reference to a single text can be made when the question is who is to be listened to as a "scientist" speaking for "science." But, to select one piece of evidence, we might go to a striking paragraph in the historian of science B. J. Teeter Dobbs's second book on the unpublished manuscripts of Isaac Newton, *The Janus Faces of Genius,*[7] her study of Newton's alchemical manuscripts that may be representative if not part of the development of modern chemical thought. Dobbs's comments are striking because of their candor, serious because of the care and seriousness of her historical work.

She remarks how long ago she began the book and goes on to explain why the work took so long, and to issue an apology. But her apology looks in a rather different direction from the apology that Lewis Thomas is making at just the same time to his "scientist friends." "My slow recognition," she writes, "that alchemical studies held religious significance for Newton himself was one of the turning points in my thinking that led me on to quite a different book. Sixteen years ago I was imperfectly detached from modernist convictions and from our general cultural perception of Newton as the founder of modern science." She says, "I was willing to entertain the heretical notion that Newton's alchemy was worthy of scholarly examination," and this is part of Dobbs's distinction today: the suppression of Newton's box of theological and alchemical papers by each generation since the seventeenth century, and the refusal to receive them as a gift, by Cambridge, Harvard, Yale, and Princeton, even though Einstein sought to be helpful, is a story in itself.[8] But, she notes, "I was not willing to entertain a religious interpretation of it."

Dobbs focuses on her own will, and her responsibility for it. She suggests that today "religious sentiments are both more acceptable and more perceptible," and she then continues, "I have apologized above for my previous attitude to Mary S. Churchill, of whose argument for the religious significance of Newton's alchemy I was at one time quite dismissive. My specific retraction may be found in Chapter 1, but this entire book may also be considered in that light." (pp. 250–51)

It is Dobbs's combined reference to modernist "convictions" and the question of separation or not from them, and to herself as earlier "quite dismissive," that evokes the atmosphere in which we work, teach, and talk today. But, of course, there is something else represented by Dobbs, the capacity to be open to evidence—the empirical spirit itself—and the possibility of being candid with and about oneself. Beside the danger of oppression and self-oppression, to which Lewis Thomas's timidity testifies, there is also hope that escape is possible.

"Newton was not a skeptic," Dobbs observes, "and in fact his assumption of the unity of Truth constituted one answer to the problem of skepticism. Not only did Newton respect the idea that Truth was accessible to the human mind, . . . he was very much inclined to accord to several systems of thought the right to claim access to some aspect of the Truth. . . . The mechanical philosophy was one system among many that Newton thought to be capable of yielding at least a partial Truth. Blinded by the brilliance of the laws of motion, the laws of optics, the calculus, the concept of universal gravitation, the rigorous experimentation, the methodological success, we have seldom wondered whether the discovery of the laws of nature was all Newton had in mind." (pp. 11–12)

The thought *that* we can wonder, and (if we examine ourselves, open to the evidence we ourselves present) that *we* do wonder, is the source of hope.

CANDOR

Return to the case of Lewis Thomas for illustration. Thomas recites the language of "emergent properties," but then he backslides. Reading Thomas one might even suppose that he recites with his fingers crossed behind his back. After he has leveled the accusation against himself that in seeing a greater mind he is proposing something mystical, something that is in charge, he says "not a bit of it." Then he says, immediately, "or maybe only a little bit." Then, realizing how devastating to a total theory "only a little bit" would be, he uses the word "fantasy" two words later to refer to his perception. Quickly he says that what he would propose is "merely." It is "unconcerned." It is a *"result,* not at all the cause" of the earth's life. It only contemplates, as might the scientific mind be so described once it had succeeded in understanding everything, since there would be nothing else to do but look at the process and oneself as part of the process looking at the process.

Then come these last sentences, of his last book. "In any case," he says making a joke—but we know that jokes are telling—"in any case," that greater mind "hasn't noticed you," you "my scientist friends." "And anyway," he continues, "if It"—he capitalizes "it," smiling no doubt at his friends' hostility that he had noted before to anything smacking of deity—"if It has a preoccupation with any part of Itself in particular, this would likely be, as Haldane once remarked, all the various and multitudinous beetles." The words at the end, the last words, have to do with concern; they are a projection of the existence, in the world, of concern.

Thomas frequently escapes with a joke, jokes being the freedom of the oppressed. At the end of a chapter in which he advances a genetically grounded instinct for sensing an obligation to the well-being of one another, he observes that bees and ants are better at sensing and fulfilling the obligation than we are, and he looks forward to "better breeding" as our evolution proceeds over long stretches of evolutionary time. He notes that viruses speed the evolution of microbes by transporting bits of DNA among them, wonders whether the viruses that make us sick might be "taking hold of useful items of genetic news from time to time, then passing these along for the future of the race," and concludes: "It makes a cheerful footnote anyway: next time you feel a cold coming on, reflect on the possibility that you may be giving a small boost to evolution." (pp. 26–27) We are supposed to smile. We do smile.

But there is a problem. Why should we be interested in the species? Why this cheerfulness during a cold? Why not let genetic selection take care of that interest in the species, "our" species? Why is he *arguing* to us about obligation, with evolution toward cooperative altruism as only a backstop? If his argument is programmed, why should we listen to it? And if *listening to argument* is programmed and selected for, why not let programs do the listening? Thomas knows "obligation" is a term, a legal term indeed, that has no place in scientific thought, any more than the terms that he himself has noted have no place, "purpose," "morality," "progress." (p. 29) But he uses *obligation,* and ends with cheer.

Looking to the state of the planet after deforestation or exposure to ultraviolet light through elimination of ozone protection, or after the cold night following a thermonuclear holocaust, Thomas admits there will still be systems we call "living." But "the planet would be back where things stood a billion years ago, with no way of predicting the future course of evolution beyond a high probability that, given the random nature of evolution, nothing quite like us would ever turn up again." (p. 122) And this is an argument, made to "us," against the environmental and ecological changes our twenty-first-century powers can bring about.

Why is this an argument? Why should we care whether "nothing quite like us" would ever turn up again?

If "we" *would* turn up again, then there is no reason not to play with our powers. It makes no difference. Time is nothing in the larger view of process. We tire ourselves today to the point of exhaustion—we awake refreshed tomorrow. We hay the field—there is a second cutting. Take it: there is more where that came from. A billion years is neither short nor long. There is no "short" nor "long" where mere systems are involved. The difference between one hundred years and one billion years is only a difference of number, only a difference as 0 is different from 1. "Short" and "long" require evaluation, judgment, value, someone to whom the difference matters. Mere systems have all the time in the world.

But suppose, with Thomas, that since we are a random product of natural systems, what will appear after a billion years will not likely be "like us." Could that be a reason not to play now, for us who exist now? A reason not to do what we are moved to do, clear-cut rain forests to feed our immediate children, or extract oil so that we can be fast and mobile, or refrigerate our food with ozone-depleting gases, or take atomic risk with the planet to avoid coming under the tyranny of rulers (who like Thomas's "scientist friends" may profess to have no place for value in their minds), which we might think would be a fate worse than death, our own death or even the death of all?

Why should we care at all about the nature of some distant system within its environment as its environment then will be? If we are the random product of a billion years of evolution, and the system does not "see fit" (though those would be forbidden words) to bring forth a product "like us" in another billion years, what concern is that of ours? The dice roll six, the dice roll two. The six does not care whether a two or a six is rolled next. The dice themselves do not care. Only if there is some identification with future creatures, creatures after our individual death, creatures after the passing of every body that is in material existence at the time of our own death, identification, real, through a connection other than near succession in time in the products of the processes of the material world, can there be any claim of the distant future on our present desires.

This is part of the dilemma and difficulty seen by lawyers in bringing the criminal law to bear in environmental matters, first legislatively, then judicially in administering criminal environmental laws. In either setting, the value being celebrated by environmental law must be expressed and faced if there is to be punishment for crime. Juries will encounter it and the problem in it increasingly in environmental law and argument, that same environmental law to which Thomas anxiously looked and others like him turn today whom he would include in the "no more than a million or so genuine scientists in the earth's population."9

But the problem now seen in this environmental guise is not an unfamiliar one: it is also the fundamental problem of democracy, the identification of one individual with another to the point that sacrifice is willing, or respect for the vote of another is real. To extend democracy beyond the tribe and the state, ultimately to the entire world, is to uncover the secret dependence of democracy on spiritual brotherhood and sisterhood: the dependence of liberty upon equality, and of equality upon fraternity, fraternity, which a leaf does not have with another leaf, nor a whirlpool with another whirlpool, nor an equation with another equation, nor any system with what is only another system.

Back and forth Thomas goes. Language for his "fragile species" is at one point in his discussion "the property of language," a trait. (pp. 160–61) Seen evolutionarily, it is at an early stage, "just beginning to emerge and evolve as a useful trait." It is a "genetically determined gift, no doubt about it," a "result"—the word he echoes in his apology to "science" at the end. "What holds us together in interdependent communities is language, for which we are almost certainly as programmed by our genomes as songbirds are for birdsong."

(p. 80) "Surely," he says, "we are dominated by genes for language, hence for culture itself" (p. 123), as he seeks to bridge the difference between "sociobiologists" and the "antisociobiology faction" who are arguing over whether human altruism is "genetically governed" or whether, instead, "behavior" of this kind is attributable "solely to cultural influences."

Language, reified, a thing, is an emergent property,[10] "so complex and intricate a mechanism." (p. 164) But this is Lewis Thomas, my own Lewis Thomas whose voice I have appreciated over so many years. His style is his own, his meaning is his own. For him language produces "an indisputable singular, unique self" (p. 18), and even a song sparrow's song "becomes his own, particular, self-specific song." (p. 24) "Whatever happened in the human brain to make this talent for language a possibility remains a mystery," he writes. And after that word "mystery," and after an hour of his pages and his voice and his use of language, the suggested explanation he sets against this mystery, the explanation which is alone allowed if it is to be explicit, is almost comically ragged and poor—"a new set of instructions in our DNA for the construction of a new kind of center" or "a more general list of specifications." (p. 24)

Despite himself his language of which he displays such a love in his practice, his language which is our language, leads him to that despised entity, the individual, that thorn in the side of those for whom the only allowable kind of mind is, as he recites at the end (p. 192), "unconcerned with the details." We may remember the Rabbis' one thing—"in the entire created universe there is only one thing of absolute value, . . . the human individual."[11] We may wonder whether in a mind so richly stocked as Thomas's there was not some awareness that "a mind unconcerned with the details," which should not worry his "scientist friends," was playing off "God is in the details." This is the Lewis Thomas who knows that "we are the anomalies for the moment" in a Nature marked by cooperation. "We are different, to be sure, but not so much because of our brains as because of our discomfiture, mostly with each other."[12] (p. 25) These "each other" are present to his mind.

This is the Lewis Thomas too who knows metaphor well, who uses metaphor. He is inclined to compare words to genes (rather as the physicist Stephen Hawking finds it natural to equate words with units of heat in his *Brief History of Time*).[13] If, in "several different languages, you can find consistent similarities between certain words of those languages, you are permitted to deduce that another word, parental to all the rest, existed at some time in the past in an earlier language. It is the same technique as is now used by today's molecular biologists for tracking back to the origin of today's genes. . . . For the molecular geneticists, a theoretical species called the 'U-bacteria,' speaking in ancient but still recognizable biochemical words, serves the same function. . . ." (p. 162) But then the poet in him is drawn to make his first example of the use of language, the cocktail party in which human beings using words are using them to mean something entirely different from the meaning they are statistically "normally" used to convey.

Thomas knows. Over and over he tells he knows, indirectly and semiconsciously, or directly, that there is not only the question "how," but the question "why." "Why is being being; why not nonbeing?" he asks. "Why should there be something, instead of nothing? How do you organize a life, or a society, in accordance with physical laws that forbid purpose, causality, morality, and progress, especially when you have to do so with brains that stand alive with these very notions?" (p. 29) He argues that "the experience that is above all others in its importance for the modeling of a young child's mind is, in my view, a combination of affection and respect . . . this magical formula" (pp. 62–63), knowing full well that this "respect" simply does not figure and is without meaning in a self-regulating system that is merely there.

Respect is no more there than it would be in a system of law if law were merely a system that is merely there, a system of rules like the rules that are conceived to produce "emergent properties." Thomas wants to use the description "amiable" for a living Nature marked by cooperation and self-restraint (pp. 34, 159), a Nature not "mean" as "economic man" is mean, *homo economicus* the premise and goal of a properly functioning fully competitive microeconomic system. He wants to counter human fear of Nature "red in tooth and claw," late-nineteenth-century Nature. But he must say— thinks he must say—thinks he knows—would say he knows—that late-twentieth-century Nature has no place for amiability either, any more than it has a place for meanness.

Just as he wants to argue obligation, and does argue obligation, as he appeals to us with all his eloquence to recognize obligation to the least fortunate, to the distant future, to the lovely earth—but is not allowed to contemplate in any open way a working world in which obligation would have any place or meaning—so he argues against drug addiction on the ground that it is a "trick," "artificial," that interferes with and "meddles" with "reality," with authentic experience which should receive the respect anything authentically human should receive. (p. 36)

But he knows he is also transgressing. As he goes on to discuss various kinds of drug addiction, he treads carefully. He says "I suppose" that these dilemmas all share origins of "some sort" in defects in the "moral fiber" of people, "whatever that may mean." "Something" has "gone wrong," and the cost of "that something, whatever it is," cannot "of course be measured only in dollars." (p. 58) "Of some sort," "whatever that may mean," "something," "whatever it is," are little nods back to those frowning at the moral dilemma, at the use of the word "wrong," at the very notion of the "artificial."

Thomas knows, but is suspended. "If I had the responsibility for putting together a closed ecosystem as huge as the one on this planet, with the intention of having it persist and survive by evolution, I would put this one property in at the very beginning." (pp. 34–37) That "property" is "pleasure in being alive."

Put this in, he says, "as a basic property of everything alive, excluding it from natural selection and any sort of competition, violating all the rules but never mind. Never mind the rules in this single case, make an exception here, allow for the pure fun that ravens have swooping down in the winds along the sides of mountain cliffs, allow for what cats do when not busy with serious cat business, make a provision for humans, especially young children playing, put in a mechanism that can handle the inside of the messages conveyed both by the Fourteenth Quartet and the fourth movement of the *Missa Solemnis*, where the violin and the human voice suddenly turn into a single voice, and install the receptor for that word in that line of that poem, that jolt of that image. Take into account the need of an organism to know, for sure, that it is alive. In short, make the game worth playing, for all the players."

Thomas knows that the game is not worth playing, he suspects it would not be played, without something that "violates the rules," those wonderfully reified *rules* his friends insist upon. Put in a "mechanism," yes, but one that "can handle the inside" of messages. Install a "receptor," yes, but for a word in a line of a poem.

Music, art, language are there before him, and he holds onto them, pulls them inside, knows they have an inside and not only an outside. But he cannot let go of the clanking language of "mechanism" and "receptor," as out of place in his paragraph as spurs in a double bed. "Never mind . . . " "Make an exception . . . " "Allow for . . . " "Put in . . . " "Take into account . . . " To whom is he speaking, appealing? When he looks back over his own memories he says he finds that most of them are "remembrances of other people's thoughts, . . . metamemories," and that a "surprising number turn out to be wishes rather than recollections, hopes that the place really did work the way everyone said it was supposed to work, hankerings that the one thing leading to another has a direction of some kind, and a hope for a pattern from the jumble, an epiphany out of entropy." (p. 17) He implies that these are only wishes, doomed hopes, his equation of a "pattern" with an "epiphany" being an expression of the doom. An epiphany, as Joyce so nicely puts it, is the sudden realization of the whatness of a thing. "Pattern" is in the world of form, whatness is in the world of substance. Making an epiphany a *mere* "pattern," not different from dead branches he sees against the sky, is renouncing substance, as he feels he must.

He turns from this to begin the work of his book, to show to human beings, his audience, that the cell, the individual, and the earth are of a piece. He comes to the end, and does not know what safely to do with the whole. For there is an emptiness in the "news" he has constantly coursing into the mechanism that senses pleasure in living, which he would suspend the rules to insert in everything alive. "What could it be, then, this news? . . . " "It must be something important," he says. It turns out to be only the news of being alive, but, still, "it must be something important." And empty of substance the "contemplation" which, at the end, is all he can explicitly allow the great mind he perceives in the whole.

Thomas's professed vision of the nature of the world that includes us, Thomas's picture of everything when everything is included, we know is inadequate, incoherent, and wrong. We know that, that at the least, even if we could not do better than he in presenting a picture that is adequate, coherent, and right.

How do we know? Do we just know, like a stubborn child, that his vision does not fit the truth?

Some of us know, and report in ways that compel our attention, from art and through art, from music and through music, from direct touch of expressed meaning. Revelation some call it: a true epiphany, which candor with ourselves and with others allows through, as more than a wish or a hope.

Less direct, more inferential, we know from a sense of necessity as strong as the necessity we feel in gravity itself.

And we know from Thomas, because Thomas tells us so in so many ways.

Chapter Three

EVERYTHING, ONLY, AND NOTHING BUT

Let us turn from Lewis Thomas to the sources of the pressure upon him, that he feels and speaks of in his last work.

The principal testimony we will use in these next chapters is a set of recorded conversations on mind, matter, and mathematics between a neurobiologist and a mathematician, both well known and much honored. In any reading of belief it will be important to particularize.

Of course with particularization comes the question of the representativeness of what is read. I hope we will see and agree that in the matter of science and cosmology the very presence of that question is part of the evidence of what is actually believed by any of those we might choose to read.

But, first, we may return to a passage from a contemporary philosopher also well known and widely read, John Searle. It was partially set out in the first of the columns with which we began, of twentieth-century accounts of the nature of things. Philosophy such as this of Searle's is a step removed from actual scientific work, which work we know has preceded any credal test and in its highest forms may indeed be driven by love and awe. But urgings such as Searle's—for philosophy is more than idle speculation—are a step closer to the human consequences of adoption and enforcement of the views Thomas ascribes to "science" and his "scientist friends." The passage is from Searle's *The Rediscovery of the Mind*,[1] published in the last decade of the century at about the same time as Thomas's *Fragile Species* and Dobbs's study of Newton. It was widely reviewed and favorably noticed:

> It goes without saying that our "scientific" world view is extremely complex and includes all of our generally accepted theories about what sort of place the universe is and how it works. . . . Some features of this world view are very tentative, others well established. At least two features of it are so fundamental and so well established as to be no longer optional for reasonably well-educated citizens of the present era; indeed they are in large part constitutive of the modern world view. These are the atomic theory of matter and the evolutionary theory of biology. Of course, like any other theory, they might be refuted by further investigation; but at present the evidence is so overwhelming that they are not simply up for grabs. . . .
>
> Basic to our world view is the idea that human beings and other higher animals are part of the biological order like any other organisms. Humans are continuous with the rest of nature. But if so, the biologically specific characteristics of these animals—such as their possession of a rich system of consciousness, as well as their greater intelligence, their capacity for language, their capacity for extremely fine perceptual discriminations, their capacity for rational thought, etc.—are biological phenomena like any other biological phenomena. Furthermore, these features are all phenotypes. They are as much the result of biological evolution as any other phenotype. . . . [M]any thinkers whose opinions I respect, most notably Wittgenstein, regard it as in varying degrees repulsive, degrading, and disgusting. . . . But, like it or not, it is the world view we have. Given what we know about the details of the world . . . this world view is not an option. It is not simply up for grabs along with a lot of competing world views. Our

problem is not that somehow we have failed to come up with
a convincing proof of the existence of God or that the hypothesis of an afterlife remains in serious doubt, it is rather that in
our deepest reflections we cannot take such opinions seriously.
When we encounter people who claim to believe such things,
we may envy them the comfort and security they claim to de-
rive from these beliefs, but at bottom we remain convinced
that either they have not heard the news or they are in the
grip of faith. . . . When I lectured on the mind-body problem
in India and was assured by several members of my audience
that my views must be mistaken, because they personally had
existed in their earlier lives as frogs or elephants, etc., I did
not think, "Here is evidence for an alternative world view," or
even "Who knows, perhaps they are right." And my insensi-
tivity was much more than mere cultural provincialism: Given
what I know about how the world works, I could not regard
their views as serious candidates for truth.

In taking this one text we do Searle something of the same dis-
service he does his Hindu respondents. Searle is known for his in-
sistence in public debate on the difference between understanding a
language and machine manipulation of the sounds and forms of a language. It could be possible, taking Searle's written work as a whole,
and without going on to his life, to find indications of lack of convic-
tion. But while in Lewis Thomas such indications abound, on a page,
in a paragraph, even within a sentence, they do not abound here, and
this passage I think is representative of the sources beyond Searle of
the sense of what "science" is that evokes the response "antiscience."

TOTAL THEORY AS ACHIEVEMENT OR OBJECTIVE

This is a statement, succinct and straightforward, of what we
have called total theory. To play with definitions, it is theory because
it introduces or assumes a particular form of thought, theory because
it requires discussion and persuasion as other experiences may not,
theory because it offers to predict, perhaps control, "explains" as is

said. It is total because it circles back and explains itself and its genesis. It explains the theorist proposing the theory as well as those to whom the theory is proposed. A total theory reaches out to explain challenges to the theory, to explain even the very language in which the theory is expressed and urged, and, as may appear, believed. With nothing outside it, nothing partial about it, with those who think, talk, and argue about it included within its terms, it is ultimate, final, closed.

Academic or nonacademic, most know when they are personally or vicariously in the vicinity of a theory that is a "theory of everything," or total. It will be remembered how objections to Freudian explanation became the clinical condition of "resistance" to Freudian explanation. Challenge to the conspiracy theories of nineteenth-century anti-Semitism only showed that the challenger was part of the conspiracy. Opposition to Maoist theory was evidence of the truth of "Maoism" and provided grounds for the elimination of the objector. These and the like are part of common lore, sources of dark jokes easily caught; and caught in them is the flavor if not the essence of total theory.

A cosmology of totalizing theory has a recognizable pattern whether it is presented as a present necessity—sole option for anyone who has heard the news—or as an animating ideal. Searle suggests the time of total theory is with us. Others look forward to it, putting it as what there is to yearn for and to try for. An end-of-century symposium on the brain from the American Academy of Arts and Sciences begins, "In contemporary science, two vast and exciting areas have opened up in this century: one involves cosmology . . . and the other, all that relates to interior man. . . . " A quotation from Isaiah Berlin is set out to describe the goal, without irony, though Berlin's life work was seeking the origins of the total, in all its twentieth-century expressions: "'The ideal of all natural science is a system of propositions so general, so comprehensive, connected with each other by logical links so unambiguous and direct that the result resembles as closely as possible a deductive system, where one can travel along wholly reliable routes from any point on the system to any other.'" "Certainly," it is said, "the ideal of brain science shares these goals."[2]

Even Oliver Sacks, so known for his openness and interest in the individuality of patients with neurological deficits, finds the Nobelist and neuroscientist Gerald Edelman's "ideas extremely exciting, providing a neural basis as they aim to do, for the entire range of mental processes from perception to consciousness, and for what it means to be human and a self."[3] The neuroscientist Steven Rose, also looking to the next century of work, concludes that "we neuroscientists lack, and badly need . . . some overarching theory of brain and mind. . . . Much of neuroscience, psychology and indeed the philosophy of mind is still stuck in a Cartesian mould, not so much that of dualism as that of insisting on the isolation of the individual as a thinking monad, instead of being part of a process which indissolubly locates people in time and space, as products of evolution, development, social and personal history, in continued interaction with their physical and social environment. It is to achieve that much deeper integration which must be the real task of the sciences of the twenty-first century."[4]

There is work to be done, years but not so very many, before the world envisioned unfolds to fill every corner of the mind. But the elements of the world envisioned are with us already, both the presences and the absences: the swirl of process, the pause of system; the absence of purpose and spirit, the absence of person and individual, the absence of transcendence of time or type. In that part of what the theorist says in which he is talking in this way, the tone (again, in this part of what he says) is not one of speculation or wonderment, or doubt about visions that fail to extend to "all" or "the entire range" of human reality. Though the details have not been grasped, nor perhaps the very outlines of their interaction, the "alls," "everythings," "nothing buts" are in place. The "musts" in the descriptions point to the reality of the desired as to a world over the horizon: the cognitive neurologist Semir Zeki concludes a discussion of beauty—we may note his "all" and "must obey"—"Aesthetics, like all other human activities, must obey the rules of the brain, of whose activity it is a product. . . ."[5] And even the possibility that full grasping may be beyond human capacity, despite desire and drive, is itself drawn into the vision, to be explained, rather as in totalitarian social and political theory dissent is drawn in to be explained.

THE TONE OF TOTAL THEORY

Return once more to Searle's summary statement of total theory, total theory that is presented as with us now. One aspect of it we should note is the reflection of the language of "property" pervasive in mathematics, philosophy, and the sciences, in Searle's "features," "characteristics," and "phenotypes." Held out as if grasped in the hand are intelligence, consciousness, and language. Second, and associated with the first, is the disappearance of the individual, or, in Lewis Thomas's word, "unconcern" for the individual, a well-known aspect also of twentieth-century totalitarian thought in social and political matters. Searle's signal of this is the word "phenotypic," which makes intelligence or language part of a system in which the transient units are fungible, rather than an experience or phenomenon of which an individual speaks with special if not ultimate authority, which indeed (this intelligence, this language) an individual speaks and does not just speak of.

Third is the pervasive use of "we" and "our" which does not include all of us, or all of us who are not demented or impaired, or in fact the majority or the great majority of us, but is rather very much a constructed "we," like the "we" used by the nineteenth-century English in India but less natural than that, covering a running and sometimes bitter argument about who is to be counted in and who is out, whose views matter and whose do not, who speaks authoritatively for "us" and who cannot or does not.

Finally, there is the dismissiveness of the tone, the attitude that Dobbs apologized for in herself, which is illustrated here by Searle's unembarrassed telling of his reaction to his Indian interlocutors, his rejection of their testimony about themselves as evidence, his unwillingness to even begin to translate what was being said to him in an effort to understand. His move is to explain rather than listen, the closure of his mind reflecting the closed system of thought characteristic of total theories, with no place for any opening out to the person and the personal. "We remain convinced," he says, that "they have not heard the news"—the "news," half-conscious wordplay on Searle's part perhaps, as there was perhaps play by Thomas on "God is in the details." Spreading the Gospel meant spreading the "good news." This is the news that replaces the Gospel. But this is not good news. Searle knows it, and might be taken to enjoy it after a fashion.

This fourth aspect, tone, attitude, is not itself to be dismissed. Style and substance may not be the same, but they cross, each drawing on and implied by the other. What may fairly be called ugliness is often perceptible in the pressing of total theory. Joseph Weizenbaum, a pioneer in computer programming, has noted it in the specific context of discussions within and about cognitive science.[6] Searle is more blithe than ugly, despite his description of Hinduism and Buddhism, and it is certainly true that mathematicians excited by a breakthrough at last, or playing music—when I was young and in a nonmusical town, it was the mathematicians who played music together—generally do not introduce it. The writing of Newton, or Darwin, or Einstein does not raise the thought of it. Freud even in his polemical aspect, Freud who pressed hard toward total theory and evoked strong responses, does not—and retranslation of Freud's German may pull Freud still further from it.[7] But ugliness is to be seen now, in the arguments and polemics of the late twentieth century.

It cannot be discounted as a source of antiscience. The more it is seen or found, the more it may also say something about the problem of total theory itself. It was, after all, so often remarked in descriptions of the impression made by fascism as a whole, the gestalt of it, when coming upon it as a phenomenon, fresh, that there was an ugliness about it, a crudeness, that interfered with its seductiveness, seductive though it was. Systematic anti-Semitism, for instance in its nineteenth-century form, could be ugly even for those not immediately affected by it: not just threatening, but ugly. Ugliness has been a feature much remarked upon in twentieth-century Eastern European and Russian communism—Eastern European literature is replete with references to it. The same is said of forms of modern architecture and urban planning, of forms of capitalism and of its economic theory. And when ugliness is remarked upon, in these contexts, even professed aesthetic relativists may find themselves agreeing despite themselves.

Respect and Disrespect

The use of "ugly" is a pointing to something and ought not, if listened for, be heard as the mere expression of disagreement. There are two aspects to what may call it to mind. One is disrespect, the other dislike. Disrespect and dislike often run together, but they need not. They lie on either side of the distinction between inaction and action—such as it is: legal analysis has great difficulty with the difference when working with responsible decision making. The distinction here is that between what tends in its degrees toward cold indifference, and what tends in its degrees toward positive hatred.

For the first aspect, disrespect, we may go back to Lewis Thomas, who has no animus, in fact, quite the reverse. In his review of the neurobiological literature leading to his proposal that there is something within the brain that "makes the game worth playing," his proposal that the something is a capacity to experience pleasure in living, and his conclusion that it is of such importance that he would exclude it "from natural selection" and suspend "the rules" to have it (*Fragile Species,* pp. 35–36), he comments: "Granted, this is a distorting, terribly unnatural, fundamentally misleading way for it to be revealed to us, by so artefactual a system for demonstrating its existence. There is something distasteful, even nasty, about viewing a rat nearly killing himself by stimulating a part of his brain that gives him ineffable pleasure. But pass that. . . ." (p. 34) And he goes on from rats to ravens swooping, cats playing, and then to the human being listening to music.

Later, in describing the origin and mechanism of the "property" of language, Thomas discusses the song sparrow and "his elaborate song, stereotyped in its general message but ornamented by himself alone. . . . If deafened as a nestling, he will sing nothing beyond a kind of buzz. The cells responsible for the song of a canary are typical, conventional-looking neurons, easily recognized in stained sections of the brain. . . ." (pp. 160–61) Then, from the "childhood" of the song sparrow, he moves to the yet unplumbed mysteries of how children acquire language and with such ease. (p. 170)

Given this characterization of language, as a property of a system, a property of what must be inside the skull of a creature that looks like a human being, what is the answer to a proposal that a child be treated like a young song sparrow? One or more deafened, one or more kept in silence, one or more sacrificed from time to time and its brain sliced and stained? Mid-twentieth-century experiments on human beings anyone can see being performed, preserved on monitors running in the Holocaust Memorial Museum.[8] The answer that child and song sparrow are very different is not explicitly available. The single vision has been expressed too many times, that, in Searle's words, humans are continuous with the rest of nature, and nature can be nothing more than a system.

Thomas saw what we do even to the rat as "nasty." But he justified it, by the wonder that it revealed. (p. 34) What is striking in much discussion of total theory now is that it is not a *wonder* that is sought to be revealed, but a further and further relished demonstration that we and our responsibility—the burden of our consciousness and sense of being—do not really exist. Insofar as justification is thought necessary at all, nastiness not being strictly admissible within the theory, the justifications advanced do not justify. There is, expressed in one way or another, a squirming at the idea of justification.

We are protected from what we do to animals, today, when we think we no longer think of sacrifice and union, by seeing animals rather as machines; but then in the background is the proposal that we see ourselves as the same. The membrane between the rat or the sparrow, and the child, becomes very thin. And the answers to the question, "Why not the child?" are not convincing.

If this be indeed what being a scientist must be (which the scientist in each of us may doubt), the scientist is hiding something. The sense of dealing with a dissembler is perhaps part of the unattractiveness of the situation. But the hiding suggests worse than a lack of belief in what is being said. It suggests, here, a belief most hard for the questioner asking "Why not the child?" to believe is a belief. It tends to lead the questioner to seek an *explanation* for the saying of it rather than treating it as a *proposal* made to her: belief that there is really no more reason to refrain from puncturing out an eardrum of a child than from puncturing out an eardrum of a song sparrow, and, certainly, no reason to hesitate with a sparrow.

For this, after the experience of the twentieth century, has a special ring to it, a summoning up of intersections between total theory of a cosmological kind and the earthbound totalitarian in social and political thought. The question of cruelty, like the question of respect, does not arise when human beings are seen as things, ingredients of systems, fungible units. The "logs" in cages, the children stamped with the same number as the guinea pigs beside them, the death camps, the gulags, the induced famines, the killing fields: the rational administration of suffering and death in the twentieth century differs with a gnawing difference from the horrors of earlier centuries, and sits with us today. Joseph Weizenbaum remarked of a colleague's comment "the brain is merely a meat machine," that the choice of the word "meat" rather than "flesh" was "a very deliberate choice of words that clearly testifies to a kind of disdain of the human being." So too the celebrated aphorism in physiology, "the brain secretes thought as the liver does bile," testifies as much to its utterer's attitude toward thought when he speaks, as to the nature of thought. "Meat," Weizenbaum pointed out, "is dead, can be burned or eaten, can be thrown away; whereas flesh is living flesh, and a certain sense of dignity is associated with it. . . . [I]f we talk about burning flesh, it is a horror image. Why . . . say 'meat machine' and not flesh machine?" When Weizenbaum made the point in a public meeting, his colleague Daniel Dennett, he says, stood up and said, "If we are to make further progress in Artificial Intelligence, we have to give up our awe of living things."

"An absolutely incredible statement," Weizenbaum commented, "but not to the Artificial Intelligence community." "We have seen that such scientific ideas—speaking about modern science—enter the public consciousness very quickly and help to build a world picture, a *Weltanschauung,* of the general public, of people who have no idea where these things come from, and have very serious consequences in political and cultural life. . . . An example, which is not scientific, although it owes something to modern science: the idea that some human beings are vermin and therefore not worthy of living as human beings. That idea made the Holocaust possible. It would have been impossible without such an idea. . . . What this worldview does is present a picture of what it means to be a human being, which allows us to deal with human beings in a way that I think we ought not to—to kill them, for example."[9]

Statements and positions about the nature of the human being, believed or not believed, do have a different quality at the end of the twentieth century than at the end of the nineteenth century. After the eugenics of the early part of the twentieth century in the United States, and in Germany in the 1930s and 1940s, a comment in 1970 by a most distinguished French geneticist, "There is nothing to prevent immediate application to human beings of the selection processes used for race-horses, laboratory mice or milch cows. But it seems desirable to know first the genetic factors involved in such complex qualities as originality, beauty or physical endurance," is no longer the bold and shibboleth-smashing thrust it might once have been.[10] Such indifference to the century's history as implies an acceptance, moves toward ugliness.

But it is also possible and more than possible that when the answers of a scientist to the question "Why *not* deafen the child like the song sparrow?" do not convince and leave an impression that the scientist is hiding something, what the scientist may be hiding is an actual belief that there is a difference between the child and the song sparrow, even that the deafening of the song sparrow must be truly justified. There is not disdain.

DISLIKE

The second aspect of the ugliness perceptible in description, discussion, and urging of total theory is its positive aspect, the animating drive in it, to attack, extirpate, destroy, to win and to occupy the field alone. There is, sadly, animus to be found in some of those who are thought representative and who are much honored during their lifetimes, animus that displays the heat of small hatreds rather than the coldness of indifference. It is accompanied by suspicion, a jealous watchfulness against backsliding or dissent among those who are together in the venture. The tone is such that if it were directed at them in equal measure we might predict it would cause them to cry out and seek the aid of force to smooth their way.

Remarkable, interesting in itself, is the fact this tone and the frequency with which it is encountered are not more noticed and commented upon. It is more than rough talk, or the occasional discourtesies of strong argument. The Nobelist Jacques Monod's *Chance and Necessity*, a widely used statement of the total adequacy of modern biological thought (and an argument, incidentally, against "vitalists" from the physical sciences represented by Elsässer, Polanyi, and even perhaps "the great Nils Bohr himself" [pp. 27–28]), begins by offering that "the ultimate aim of the whole of science is indeed, as I believe, to clarify man's relationship to the universe." (p. xi) Monod laments, like Thomas, "the fear if not the hatred—in any case the estrangement—felt toward scientific culture by so many people today." (p. 172) He ends with a chapter that we could use to see what human candor can do, as we have used Thomas's *Fragile Species*. But in Monod's ending chapter is found, as a summation of what has been woven into the prior description and discussion, "societies of the West still teach—or pay lip-service to—a disgusting farrago of Judeo-Christian religiosity, scientistic progressism, belief in the 'natural' rights of man, and utilitarian pragmatism. The Marxist societies still profess the materialist and dialectical religion of history. . . . [A]ll these systems rooted in animism exist at odds with objective knowledge, face away from truth, and are strangers and fundamentally *hostile* to science. . . . The divorce is so great, the lie so flagrant, that it afflicts and rends the conscience of anyone provided with some element of culture, a little intelligence. . . ." (p. 171)

The Nobelist François Jacob's *The Logic of Life*, from the early 1970s like *Chance and Necessity*, takes as its epigraph a quotation from Diderot, "Do you see this egg? With it you can overthrow all the schools of theology, all the churches of the earth." *The Logic of Life* is also well known, characterized on its jacket by Lewis Thomas himself as "simply astonishing . . . a great story" and by Douglas Futuyma judged "as clear and compelling an exposition of the essence of biology and the nature of science as one could hope to read." It is a history of biology, the internal evidence of which we will also want to use to explore actual belief in the truth of total theories—so great is the contrast presented between Jacob's all-encompassing account of the biological, and his vision of the evolution of his all-encompassing account of the biological—biology itself—in which he had played a part. Passages from *The Logic of Life* are set out in chapter 1, and we can note them again here:

"[T]he way of viewing life and the human being has gradually changed," Jacob urges. "We can see how both have become subjects of research instead of revelation. (p. xi) . . . The intention of a psyche has been replaced

> by the translation of a message. The living being does indeed represent the execution of a plan, but not one conceived in any mind. It strives toward a goal, but not one chosen by any will. The aim is to prepare an identical programme for the following generation. The aim is to reproduce. An organism is merely a transition, a stage between what was and what will be. Reproduction represents both the beginning and the end, the cause and the aim. . . . With the development of experimental science, of genetics and biochemistry, it was no longer possible, except for the mystic, seriously to invoke some principle of unknown origin, an x eluding the laws of physics by its very essence, in order to account for the existence and properties of living organisms. . . . [B]iology has demonstrated that there is no metaphysical entity hidden behind the word "life." (pp. 2, 244–45, 306)

In the *Conversations on Mind, Matter, and Mathematics* between the mathematician and Fields Medalist Alain Connes and Jean-Pierre Changeux, director of the Molecular Neurobiology Laboratory of the Institute Pasteur and well known both in Europe and the United States, the comments of the neurobiologist ring with pejoratives. The mathematician is much on the defensive as he argues, from direct experience and perception, for a mathematical reality independent of and not reached by the all-encompassing theory pressed, and excites not just the neurobiologist's interest, but his suspicion of such a "reality that I believe exists independently of our Darwinian world, whose coherence and harmony are the very opposite of randomness." (p. 116) Nonetheless, in this pairing of mathematician and neurobiologist the mathematician does not stray far, and only rarely comments upon the tone. "I grant," Connes assures Changeux, as Thomas assured his "scientist friends,"

> that the brain is a tool of investigation, that it has nothing of the divine about it, that it owes nothing to any transcendence whatsoever. . . . If I were indifferent to the materialist point of view, I could easily claim that a better understanding of the physical and biological function of the brain contributes noth- ing to the understanding of the human mind. But that's not at all my position. . . . To affirm the existence of a mathematical reality independent of perception certainly doesn't amount to making a teleological claim. I wouldn't dare for a moment as- sert that such-and-such a mathematical object is evidence of any sort of finalism whatsoever. No mathematician would make such an argument! In no way, then, can my position be characterized as teleological. (pp. 26–28, 38)

That confession, as we shall see, is not enough to deflect accu- sations of theism; but the combinatorial quality of mathematical thought, the precise definition of its "objects," the substantive empti- ness of the system it discovers, are enough to allow Changeux to see in Connes a joint venturer. When the neurobiologist borrows words from Spinoza and says, "Nature proposes no end to its operations" and "all final causes are only pure fictions imagined by men," the mathematician replies, "I agree." Changeux goes on, "Nature itself has no meaning." (pp. 200–201)

And in addition to this negative—denial of purpose and mean- ing, and of transcendence of system and process (with one partial and explicit exception by Connes, mathematics, and one implicit ex- ception of unknown scope he also introduces, literature)—we see Connes driven too by a thirst for the total. (e.g., p. 206) After he resists Changeux's effort to incorporate physics, with its mathematical con- tent, into Darwinian process, grasping "time" back from Changeux, he returns to suggest Changeux's world might be absorbed into his own: "[W]e can have confidence that we shall eventually arrive at a mathematical picture of the outside world that incorporates this ge- netic component. . . . [U]nderstanding iteration also makes it possible to encode the living forms of the natural world." Changeux interposes, "And even the functioning of our brain"; Connes replies, "I hope so." (pp. 208–9)

Pejoratives are so widely distributed and so frequently encountered in these *Conversations* that there is in the end more than suggestion they may be intrinsic to the position being explored. Again, there is always a question of the representativeness of any example. But for a gauge of it, as with Jacob's *Logic of Life,* we may look at the admiration displayed in the book jacket comments, contributed by a variety of distinguished and well-known names. Even discounting for the genre, what is said is still useful as an indication: "Two brilliant minds"; "two outstanding intellects—each a leader in his field"; "two gifted individuals: a conversation that is remarkable for its erudition"; "a superb guide"; "the concluding remarks on ethics, setting out the credo of the neuroscientist, are the high point"; "an inside look at the workings of two great minds . . . not a book that narrowly focuses on mathematics or neuroscience; it is a set of deep insights."

And so: in speaking of the various moralities of the world the neurobiologist Changeux says, "Together they make up a virtual symphony of blindness and mutual intolerance. . . ." (p. 214) He speaks of "religions, which by their nature are intolerant." (p. 232) Belief, he says, is rather like a disease: "A belief may be defined as a specific state of nerve cell activity characteristic of an individual's interaction with others of his kind. . . . [T]hey can propagate from one brain to another, and spread 'infection' much as viral attacks do, suggesting comparisons with epidemics." (p. 227)

When the mathematician describes the experience of mathematical illumination striking, the neurobiologist replies, "You make me think of the mystical ecstasy of Saint Theresa of Avila." (p. 147) When earlier Connes says, "I've told you what I believe—what I strongly believe," the neurobiologist responds, "Be careful, you've just used the word 'believe' again!" (p. 39) Any position of Connes's that Changeux deems "metaphysical," or of anyone else's upon whom he comments, he calls a "prejudice" (e.g., p. 211), his own position the result of ridding oneself of "prejudices" (p. 213), "an act of self-discipline . . . by which one tries to eliminate . . . all remaining traces of transcendence" left by metaphysics. (p. 25) "No one,"

Changeux observes, "takes teleological arguments seriously any-more, at least not in biology." (p. 38)

Earlier he had observed, "[N]o one today—apart from certain religious fundamentalists—entertains the idea that evolution has unfolded with man, in all his perfection, as its final purpose." (p. 36) In discussing mathematics as a universal language, his comment is, "No one—no one who's not a religious believer at least—is going to say that the Word comes before Matter." (p. 20) And in the course of affirming that there is nothing of the divine or of purpose in mathematics, Connes contributes his own "no one": "Once a mathematical theorem has been proved . . . no one's going to doubt it any longer." (p. 34)

Referring to the "so-called higher organisms" (p. 94), and objecting to the frequent invocation of Gödel's theorem "to moderate the ambitions of neurobiologists, or even to call their approach into question . . . [or] to justify the idea that the 'human mind' will be for-ever resistant to science," Changeux repeats, "'The brain secretes thought as the liver does bile.'" (pp. 154–55) He "reemphasizes" that he wants to "avoid the term 'ideal' (*idéal*), which has a certain tele-ological, even spiritualistic connotation." (p. 190) And "assigning spe-cifically human qualities to external reality" is an idea he must "dis-miss," like Searle in India. It is a "*pensée sauvage*," the thought of the savage. As a biologist he is "relieved to realize that the idea I was try-ing to dismiss, of the physical world as a sort of interlocutor, isn't one you actually subscribe to!" (p. 200)

Dismissal and the pejorative contained in dismissal continue in the terms "amazing," "astonishing," "surprising." Referring to "no less distinguished a mathematician than Cantor" remarking that mathematics was "the creation of a God," Changeux exclaims, "It's amazing to hear serious scientists say such things." (p. 11) To Connes he says he "won't go so far as to compare your attitude" with that of "certain religious fundamentalists," but "I detect a sort of *finalism* that's surprising to find in a theoretical scientist." (p. 36) "If you call yourself a materialist," he presses Connes, then "you're obliged" to give the mathematical world "a material basis." (p. 44) At the end of their conversations, extending total theory to ethics, he remarks that "the scientist" who "wishes to remain true to himself" will be "obliged sooner or later to inquire into the natural and cultural bases of ethics." (p. 212)

THE WORLD OF HUMAN ACTION

Ugliness in both its forms, indifference and aggressiveness, is of more than explanatory importance for the late-twentieth-century phenomenon of antiscience, with acknowledgment of which Lewis Thomas and Jacques Monod each ended his own life's work. Accompanying and framing the total reaching, and framing the tone of contempt and dismissal, are references to power, power of some human beings over others. Joseph Weizenbaum notes them in the cognitive and computer sciences; any lawyer will be immediately sensitive to them.

In the last chapter of *Chance and Necessity,* Monod notes particularly the affliction his cosmological views will visit upon "all those among mankind who bear or will come to bear the responsibility for the way in which society and culture shall evolve." (pp. 171–72) Jacob, who begins with "Do you see this egg? With it you can overthrow all the schools of theology, all the churches of the earth," ends with a future in which "it will become possible to intervene in the execution of the genetic programme, or even in its structure, to correct some faults and slip in supplementary instructions. Perhaps it will also be possible to produce at will, and in as many copies as required, exact duplicates of individuals. . . ." (p. 323) For Changeux, discussing how in "generalized Darwinism" a "diversity generator" ("variability with its *random* component") might operate after the "evolutionary secularization of morality," with "Darwinian variations" of a random kind "propagated from one brain to another" and "selected at the level of the community," the units that he calls "mental representations . . . of moral prescriptions" are "finally retained in the minds of law-makers." (p. 231) And, of course, Lewis Thomas himself was seeking transfers of food, shelter, and accumulated funds to his "scientist friends" from others working and living on the planet.

If there is going to be power arrogated or acquiesced in, one would want not so much a more moral cadre (moral people can argue about what is moral), but a more attractive and trustworthy cadre. Quite enough ugliness is displayed by lawyers, politicians, and corporate executives, with quite enough falling away of trust on that account.

There is always a question of translation of the insights of those with particular gifts and faculties to others on the planet without such gifts and faculties, who, since no one has all gifts and faculties, may have something for translation in return. If some are going to take the work of others one would want more of a demonstrated capacity for translation, on both sides, with more likelihood of a willingness to attend to what is being offered on both sides. Anyone would want rulers, if rulers there are to be, not marked by animus and smallness of mind, rulers not marked by that distinctive combination recognizable in adolescent psychology, a pull toward power, motivation toward it, and away from responsibility, denial of it and closing the eyes to it. And now, as for the sort of rulers one would like to have, if rulers there are to be, there is the matter of what is newly at stake: the possibilities for suffering and loss are now so great, precisely because of the technology, the wonderful success of scientific method and mathematical thought.

PROSPECT

So, we do need to know what to think of what is presented to us as we move into the twenty-first century.

There is song we seek to understand. There is touch, and the touching. There is sight and insight. If the songbird is deafened and he cannot hear the song "as a young child," Thomas writes, then "what comes out later when he is ready for singing and mating is an unmelodious buzzing noise. This is one of the saddest tales in experimental biology." (p. 24) Rhesus monkeys are blinded in order for the experimenter to see how well they cope, and what forbearance or concern other rhesus monkeys will display.[11] Changeux expounding his total theory describes a "classic series of experiments": If "the eyelids are sutured on one side" of "a kitten or newborn monkey," the "functional specialization" in the "visual cortex of the adult animal" is greatly disturbed, very often irreversibly. In humans, the equivalent of such an experiment occurs spontaneously when, for example, a child is born with a cataract. . . . [A] visual deficit—blindness, in fact—. . . persists in the aftermath of an operation on the cataract done *following* the critical period. . . . These experiments, among many others, suggest . . . (pp. 110–11)

And the question, again, is this: Why not suture the eyelid of a child on one side? Why not drag one's heels in operating on a child's cataract? Whence the desire to prevent blindness in an individual member of a species, when an experiment is spontaneously presented to a researcher whose only *value,* as Monod says, is the advancement of explanation in the terms of this form of thought? In "generalized Darwinism," after all, at any level of organization, "elementary units or building blocks are recombined among themselves in 'blind,' random variation. . . . " (pp. 107–8)

If the mouth does not speak anything but blindness and indifference, this may be because the actual staying of the finger, that might reach to put out the eye of the child, itself speaks often enough. Just a finger, motionless in the air, can be sign enough.

Chapter Four

IDENTIFYING SCIENCE

THE PROSPECT CONTINUED

Lewis Thomas's "scientist friends," whose shadow fell across his thought: think of them. For Thomas they were set apart among those, us, the "fragile species" to whom he was speaking. "There are, I suppose, no more than a million or so genuine scientists in the earth's population,"[1] he had remarked in another moving essay a decade earlier on the nature of science, and he went on to discuss "their" behavior and the hope it offered the future of humanity as a whole.

But can we set "them" apart? Who among us might Thomas's "scientist friends" be? Known to him individually as friends from this small subset of a million or so out of the many billions of us around him, or swept expansively into the larger sense of friend, how did he recognize them? How might we? They do not really wear uniforms, a blue tunic to be picked out here in the crowd, a white coat there.

Is it this totalism heard voiced, heard by Thomas, by others, that marks "science" or the "scientist," or indeed "mathematics" or the "mathematician"? Much turns on this, what we may call the problem of identification of science or scientist. For if there is not sufficient reason to think the stance or tone of totalism is the nature or character of science, "antiscience" or fear of science may lose its object.

REPRESENTING SCIENCE

We have referred before to the representativeness of examples. Let us pause and consider it somewhat further in this chapter, so that the matter of representativeness will be with us when we return in the next chapter to the uncomfortable question of why in the modern world there might be fear and hostility to science.

One must work with particulars, and there is always the issue "Why this particular?" when one is outside a hierarchically organized offering of materials. Just counting will not do. Majority rule does not govern these matters. Representativeness necessarily rests on the general sense of things one or another of us writing or reading may have, and the general sense of things that knowledgeable and experienced friends may have; and the sense that we have, and others have whom we listen to, is in turn informed by a sense of the weight to be given to prizes and to the equivalent of office, which may enhance the care taken before speaking, but (we also know) may just enhance the frequency of opportunities to speak that someone offering material for our study has received.

Here, to borrow the language of the fields involved, there is a question of "definition." To meld it with the language of law, there is a question of the authority of a definition. The evidence presented on whether a cosmology advanced *is* that of science carries with it what we may call an internal problem. For the evidence is *always* particular, this book, that article, this person's statement, that person's statement. One must of course read particulars to judge belief or authenticity; and it may be true that ultimately of most importance to listeners is whether the person who does scientific work does believe what he seems to be saying on cosmology. But the interest of particulars does not stop here, with authenticity. The very fact that there is a question of representativeness, and that it is a particular with which any of us works when working on that question, has its own significance.

The first fact, the fact with which we in fact start: is it the atomic structure of matter? Or time? Or what time tells us about history? Or what history tells us about ourselves? It is none of these. There is something more fundamental. The first fact, with which we all start, is the fact we are more than one and, when one of us speaks, he or she is only one.

Each of us comes new into the world. Everything, every single thing and thought, is new to each one of us at some point in our lives, and we are here only a short time. We go, and then the newness begins again for others. We are spoken to, presented to, as we move through life—and we speak and present newness to others in turn—but whatever the subject, whatever is said, one who speaks is only one. Scientists and mathematicians *appeal,* do they not? Not just to nonscientists (if there be any wholly such) but to other scientists and mathematicians.

Everywhere within science there is scientist appealing to scientist, scientist invoking scientist. In the *Conversations on Mind, Matter, and Mathematics* we opened in chapter 3, neurobiologist Jean-Pierre Changeux seeks to extend the premises of evolutionary theory back to the subject matter of physics, with physical laws and constants themselves the product of evolutionary mechanisms. "It's *undeniable,*" he says, and we may note and underline some of his words, "that this reality, despite its extreme complexity, exhibits intrinsic *regularities* that the physicist discovers, represents in the form of simple equations, and states in the form of *laws.* . . .What would you say to the idea that the various regularities of the physical world might not be *anything more than* the product of the history of the universe, of an evolution that's still in the process of unfolding? It's a simple enough idea, and not in the least original. . . . [W]hy not extend a sort of Darwinian mechanism to the evolution of matter itself?" The mathematician Connes resists this extension, commenting that there would be a problem with the notion of "time." (pp. 201–2)[2] The biologist responds in part, "Your definition of time is inappropriate." (p. 205)

Now anyone experiencing time—you the reader who experiences time—could reject the "definitions" of both Changeux and Connes. Certainly when total theories are pushed forward to the phenomenon of human law—Searle, for example, saying that "the world of Supreme Court decisions and of the collapse of communism is the same world as the world of the formation of planets and of the collapse of the wave function in quantum mechanics"[3]—a lawyer could note the inadequacy of "the notion of time" carried with them.

But just here, within the world of scientific vision, there is disagreement or lack of agreement about time, argument about time, a desire and effort to persuade. To a degree there is a *need* to persuade, an absolute need of confirmation, without which, without any confirmation whatever, without confirmation indeed that reaches a certain degree, insight withers and assurance of truth fades.

One of the arguments made to persuade is an appeal to the views of others. When Jacques Monod ends his preface to *Chance and Necessity*, speaking of his work "as an avowed attempt to extract the quintessence of the molecular theory of the code" and setting forth "the ideological generalizations I have ventured to deduce from it," he observes that "these interpretations would find assent from the majority of modern biologists." With respect to their ethical and political aspect, he says, "I have the strengthening assurance of finding myself in full agreement with certain contemporary biologists whose achievements are worthy of the highest regard." (pp. xiii–xiv)

"Assent from the majority of modern biologists": Jacques Monod is not thinking here of a system, that veers and takes a direction some majority of its constituent units take. He would not determine the truth of his proffered vision by poll, or view truth as a statistical outcome. His subsequent reference to "certain contemporary biologists whose achievements are worthy of the highest regard," whose assent gives him "strengthening assurance," says that—that for him truth is not a statistical matter or the possession of the majority. In any event, before any polling for a majority or any statistical work were done, there would be a question of what persons to admit into the voting electorate or the statistical set: what the denominator is to be which will give meaning to the numerator, where the boundary is to be that will permit quantitative resolution of statistical variables. There is an unshakable question of identity, just as there is a question of Catholic identity in determining the views of the Church or of Catholics on matters as to which there is dissent, or there is a question of identity in inquiring into what one oneself should think, might think, or in fact, in the end, does think.

And, in considering science and fear of science or "antiscience" at the beginning of the twenty-first century, the question is about thought on the largest matters. Each of us does have a thought on these matters, however accessible it may be to us at any particular time, and whatever we may say to others or to ourselves at a particular time in the course of life. There is an oddness, that should be recognized, about our focus here, in its implicit assumption that someone's capacity to work with texts on topology (for example) qualifies that one to talk publicly of the nature of reality, or that training in chemistry or the physiology of nerve tissue equips someone to talk of the nature of the cosmos. Philosophers and theologians used to be the ones thought qualified to speak, to lecture indeed. The mantle has shifted, or been tugged away, and everywhere we see listening and response to speakers, the substance of whose work that provides their qualifications has rather little to do with the subject of their statements. Jacques Monod's strengthening assurance about his own ethical views is drawn from "certain contemporary biologists whose achievements are worthy of the highest regard." In these circumstances even lawyers—those who work regularly more than others with the legal form of thought—need not be shy in claiming qualifications, for there is no *a priori* reason why those whose expertise is in the writing or handling of legal texts (and their subjects) rather than texts on topology or nerve physiology (and their subjects) should be viewed as less qualified. We could as well explore what the actual view of law and lawyers is on cosmological questions. At least the substance of the texts on which their expertise is based touches upon these larger questions.

But our focus is science and antiscience. Lawyers are used to nonlawyers being antilawyer if not antilaw, while scientists and science depending on and appealing for public support are surprised and feel a greater sense of injury and threat from antiscience. And antiscience is more dangerous if it should dim the passing on of scientific habits of mind and work—law tends to reassert itself in the longings of those who abandon it.

THE INVOCATION OF OTHERS

If the question of identity is critical to the very notion of antiscience, consider scientists' own sense of identity and work with it.

"We neurobiologists," says Changeux in his *Conversations,* "can therefore take heart" (p. 159) in rejecting Gödel's theorem as a limit on understanding. He had observed earlier that Gödel's theorem was
frequently invoked, to call "their" approach into question, and to suggest that the mind will be forever resistant to "science." (p. 154) He
contemplates "the scientist" who "wishes to remain true to himself."
(p. 212) When Changeux refers to the views of a particular mathematician on the historically antagonistic relationship between mathematics and biology, Connes responds, "There's no question about
his originality as a mathematician. But it would be a mistake to regard him as a spokesman for mathematical opinion." (p. 5) The neurobiologist makes observations about "mathematicians" who remain
"mathematicians" for him "despite important differences of detail in
their cerebral organization—as opposed to that of nonmathematicians." (p. 112) Discussing the transmission of results of mathematical illumination "from one mathematician to another," he observes
that the "receiving brain must possess a particular faculty in order for
communication to take place," and the mathematician replies, "Of
course." (p. 118) The mathematician goes on to refer to the development of "mathematical talent" in the child, and of some children as
"gifted." In such exchanges as these on mathematics, it would seem
that what mathematics is, and what the mathematician is, is assumed
to be discrete and identifiable without regard to assent or persuasion.

On the other hand, Changeux is "amazed" to hear "serious scientists say such things" as are said by mathematicians speaking of
the nature of mathematics and referring to it as a creation of God.
Science, despite his wish, becomes less self-defining. For this distinguished neurobiologist, the equally distinguished mathematician and
physicist Roger Penrose engages in a form of prescientific "savage
thought," and is "not alone" in "assigning specifically human qualities
to external reality." (p. 200) The necessity of persuasion and the possibility of failure—that possibility which is implied in the necessity of
persuasion—cannot be put aside. "The idea is so fixed in your mind,"
the biologist exclaims to the mathematician "that mathematics constitutes a distinct world from the neurons and synapses and all the
rest of the machinery that makes up the brain, I wonder if it isn't a
waste of my time trying to challenge it." (p. 84)

As he goes about nonetheless trying to persuade, and simultaneously to maintain his own assurance in the event of failure, he uses against the mathematician the dissent and disagreement of other mathematicians. Challenging Connes on the question of whether the mathematician discovers a reality that consists of mathematical objects, or whether instead the mathematician creates mathematical objects, Changeux says, "But not all mathematicians share this belief." (p. 41) He has twice before taken the opportunity for a sally against belief as such, and here he refers to "this corpus whose special existence you *believe* in (as you know, I use the word 'believe' deliberately!)" (p. 41)—a practice on his part, we may note, which gives an air of oddity to this and much other late-twentieth-century writing that presses one form or another of total theory. Invoking the authority of the mathematician Poincaré and quoting him as a lawyer would quote a judge, the biologist suggests, "In mathematics the word 'exist' can have only one meaning: 'exempt from contradiction,'" and he argues to the mathematician opposite him that "even if you don't agree" with Poincaré's definition, "it's helpful." (p. 190)

Historicizing mathematics, the biologist ultimately argues for a process of selection, not different in kind from any other Darwinian process ranging from the evolution of physical law to the evolution of ethics, "that assures the integration of a new object with the 'cultural corpus' of current mathematics, which is itself the result of a sometimes quite erratic historical process of evolution." The mathematician accepts the social, if not sociological, aspect of mathematics, but maintains the existence of something beyond process, historical or social: "A new tool doesn't really acquire its social place in the mathematical world until the moment it permits us to force an opening that will reveal a small, hitherto undisclosed, unsuspected corner of the underlying archaic reality." (p. 190) The "us" is the mathematician, the "mathematical world" is the world of the mathematician. Again, "in order for these concepts to acquire common currency, even conversationally within the small community of mathematicians," they must serve this revelation: "Advances in knowledge are measured precisely by their impact on our understanding of archaic reality." (p. 191)

The biologist responds, "That's your definition. Not all mathematicians are obliged to accept it." The mathematician replies, "One sees it commonly used in mathematical practice." (p. 191) And then in using the challenge within mathematics posed by what are called "constructivists," the biologist observes, "They can't be accused of obscurantism: after all they *do* know the mathematical world. But for them that world exists only insofar as they can build it step by step." (p. 43) The mathematician, resisting, responds that the mathematical world "exists apart from us, because, as all mathematicians agree, its structure is independent of individual perception." (p. 56) "This position," the biologist says later, at once acknowledging it and seeking to blunt it, "you share with a few other mathematicians" (p. 179), and indeed the biologist might not engage in argument at all if he judged this mathematician's view, on cosmology and the totality or not of the biologist's theory, to be a view peculiar to this man alone.

THE SOCIOLOGICAL AND THE HISTORICAL

In observing this much-honored neurobiologist and this much-honored mathematician slipping thus into the sociology of science, we need not think ourselves implicitly moving to the position that science is a social construction and "nothing but" a social construction. We need not move to "historicism," the form of total theory espoused in the late twentieth century by those who do not call themselves scientists or mathematicians but rather "historians" or "social scientists" or "students of culture." If we did, we would have to ask ourselves whether, read as a whole, reasonably and closely, we really meant what we seemed to be saying.

To see as together in the world both ourselves and that of which we can be persuaded is not to embrace the relativism of truth including scientific truth. There is the scientist in all of us. We all, scientists included, depend on the testimony of others. Beginning with the person, connecting scientific insight to the person, with all that such connection acknowledges and affirms, does not dissolve scientific insight into historical process, scatter it, make it vanish. Persons speak and persons listen.

Observing the fact of differences within the mathematical community, or between the mathematical community and the scientific community, or within the scientific community, differences either on matters special to a discipline or on matters cosmological on which they choose to speak using their membership in the discipline as their special qualification to speak, does raise a question of identity; and it introduces the necessity of assent, assent in some measure, together with the implications that the necessity of assent brings to mind. But to observe the presence of assent and the possibility of dissent does not mean there is no identity to mathematics, or to science. Nor does it mean that identity, together with the view of particular truths or the nature of truth in general that is associated with identity, is only a statistical grouping in which the personal views of historically and culturally situated individuals are the only real units: which might be the view of the economist, with respect to all matters except economics.

There is such a thing as law, a phenomenon, human law—and it may be suggested that these whom we have been reading and quoting demonstrate no real understanding of human law, no more understanding than the understanding of mathematics by nonmathematicians whose ignorance they ridicule, such as the psychiatrist Lacan using topology in psychological theory. (p. 127) There is a legal form of thought, associated with the existence of human law. But within law, and well known to nonlawyers, is active argument and steady disagreement about both the nature of the phenomenon and the form of thought with which it is associated.

I rather think there is such a thing as poetry. But the sociology of poetry is easy to see. Peter Davison's *The Fading Smile*,[4] on the world of poetry in Boston after the Second World War, is a picture of groups meeting and approving or not approving a piece of writing as a poem or a good poem; admitting or not admitting to the group those proffering pieces of writing as poems; inviting or not inviting individuals to read; publishing or not publishing. Those not invited, not admitted, not published, fade from view together with what they offer as poetry—there are very few George Herberts or Thomas Chattertons. Thus the verdict on the question of what poetry is or what good poetry is, the *definition* of poetry, to use contemporary biologists' or philosophers' language that is so antithetical to the language of poetry, is "social." But none of these approving, inviting, publishing, rejecting would say that what poetry is or what makes a poem good is the vector product of their various views. If they did, they might well be denied their identity as poets.

The verdict on poetry is the verdict of a society that, to a degree almost equal to the world of mathematics, consists of those who claim or claim to recognize a special gift. Lawyers in the world of law are different in this regard, the legal form of thought more ordinary. Certainly mathematicians are a self-defining group, calling themselves by a name, and perceiving a reality (whether constructed or preexisting) that others cannot see. Attention by others to either poetry or mathematics, to the writing that is offered as poem and makes its way into publication, or to the mathematician who must translate what he sees and says if he is to be understood at all, assumes that there is substance or reality—*poetry, mathematics*—toward which this social process strives, that there is something to argue about and not simply argument, presumes perhaps the existence of the *gift*. Attention itself is evidence of the assumption: pull the assumption, and attention turns elsewhere.

There is, to be sure, an alertness to numbers, to the "no one," to the one that is "only one," to the few, the many, the majority, the "all" and "everyone." But the assent of another, then another, and then more, is viewed as confirmation and as winning a personal struggle within, as much by the one who wins as by the one who assents. Who would have more than a passing spectator's interest in the scraps among members of a street gang, however sharp their jackets? The faith is pervasive that acceptance is evidence of truth, not just evidence of acceptance. Dissent operates in the reverse fashion, and places each back on the road toward assent.

THE AUTHORITATIVE

With regard then to what "science" is, we can observe that neither totalism, nor the ugly face it can show, is universal among those who call themselves "scientists" or "mathematicians" and who are accepted as such by others who give themselves the same identity. That fact alone, of dissent within "science" or "mathematics," would put anyone, tempted or not to what Thomas calls "antiscience," to the task of deciding when it is that "science" speaks and what it is that science says about the nature of the world as a whole, the world including us and science and the scientist. And again, that determination would no more be made by looking statistically or for a majority view, than scientists or mathematicians would determine good science or good mathematics by poll.

How we are to do so, how we are to proceed, what the method (if you will) might be, we have touched upon in discussing Lewis Thomas. It is to inquire what self-identifying speakers would say if they were candid with others and with themselves—with us, indeed. It is to inquire on the basis of what they say and what they do in the world, while ourselves remembering—or believing and continuing to believe—that they are persons and individuals, living in the world, like us. I hesitate to suggest this is the method of the lawyer, so self-interested, so imperial, so counterintuitive that might seem. But it is the method of the lawyer, not by any means confined to the lawyer, but embodied and nameable in the lawyer's discipline and practice. Law has innate sensitivity to the exercise of and appeal to authority where scientists and mathematicians are speaking for and to something larger than themselves, and are appealing for deference or action on the part of others. To the judge or lawyer, theorists are witnesses, as we have said—expert witnesses, to be sure, of wonderful scope and capacity often beyond that encountered in the legal profession or elsewhere, but witnesses still. And there are many of them, and they conflict, and they succeed one another over the course of a lawyer's career on the bench or in practice. Law presumes a responsible mind at work in the testimony of witnesses, as it presumes a responsible mind behind its own texts; and much of the design of the procedures and institutions, systems indeed, through which law operates is focused upon making responsibility possible in fact. In working with testimony, law's drive is toward candor, toward the authentic, be it the authenticity of a proffered document or the authenticity of a proffered view. Its way is to look at the whole evidence, to leave nothing out, to see all that comes from the person whose testimony is evidence laid out to be examined.

Law's easy transcendence of the here and now, in its construction of law and in its work with its texts, may make it a biased judge of propositions that deny the possibility of transcendence of any kind. Its focus upon and concern for the individual may be viewed as a handicap in approaching visions, political or cosmological, which have no place for individual voice—in which individuals are fungible and dispensable, units to be decomposed or recombined into other units, and, except as systems and parts of systems, without interest and certainly without intrinsic value. But the matters that we are discussing here and that trouble so many at the beginning of the twenty-first century are not a legal case, and it is not lawyers who will judge. I suggest the affinity between law's way and how science and antiscience might be handled, simply to place it. The natural and important step is to look for candor, for authenticity and what the candid would be, and in doing so to look at the whole of the testimony that each of us presents to others, and to ourselves.

Chapter Five

THE PROBLEM OF
THE NEGATIVE

In the mid-twentieth century James Neel was a pi-
oneer investigator of the genetic effects of exposure to the atomic
bomb. He is often called the father of modern human genetics. While
he was studying the genetics of the Yanomami people in Venezuela
in 1968, he had what he called an "epiphanic experience" and wrote
of it in his 1994 autobiography, *Physician to the Gene Pool:*

> We'd made camp well up a remote tributary to the Orinoco,
> across the river from a Yanomama village. I had slung my ham-
> mock on a bluff beside the river. Slumping into it that night,
> looking off across the river with an unobstructed view of the in-
> credible richness of the tropical stars, the stars and I were sud-
> denly one. Man is forever wondering how he fits into the in-
> tricate web of life; these are the moments when he is part of
> it, free of debate between the committees of the mind. I won-
> dered at the time, and at rare moments thereafter, if this was
> evidence of some dangerous instability that might ultimately
> prevail. It's the kind of experience you don't share with your
> "hard science" friends. (pp. 188–89)

After Neel died in 2000, an extended public controversy arose over the effects of his intervention into the lives and indeed bodies of the human subjects of his study in Venezuela. Some traced his actions to what they took to be his fundamental view of the world.[1]

Neel the distinguished geneticist points like Lewis Thomas, in his thought of hiding (from his "hard science friends") such an opening out in his hammock, and he points in his concern about himself, that there was an "instability" within him that might be "dangerous" and "ultimately prevail." Certainly it is tempting to see an orthodoxy in scientific discussion of larger matters, a defining center from which an individual scientist may be more or less distant and be therefore granted more or less of a claim to be a true scientist or, in Jean-Pierre Changeux's phrase, a scientist "true to himself." It is easy to suppose that the "scientist friends" whom Thomas and Neel look at over their shoulder are dressed in a uniform which identifies them. If negation had a color, that color might be the color of such a uniform.

Then it would not be surprising if negation begat negation, the "anti" of antiscience. We ought not ignore the negative, and we may, in considering the negative as such, be pushed on toward some further understanding of our situation when presented with statements made by others about the largest things.

THE ELEMENTAL NEGATIVE

The use of the word "astonish" or "amaze" can be put down as just one of the pejoratives sprinkling late-twentieth-century discussion. But what is "astonishing" or "amazing" rather than merely "intriguing" or "interesting" can also be taken as another pointer to identity. "Astonish" steps into the realm of belief and commitment, of settled expectation and betrayal. Changeux finds it "amazing" to hear mathematicians, whom he terms "scientists," speak of divinity. Stand back, and look again at the range of discussion in the essays, books, and popularizations that appeared in such great numbers in the second half of the twentieth century: the reaching to deny spirit—and reference to "theism" as a counterdenial of scientific truth—is striking. It is constant and widespread. Anything to the contrary "amazes" and "astonishes." Even Newton and Einstein astonish.

So when one muses on what drives the writing of the book or the essay in which one is reading the urgings and the arguments, when one tries to sense where the delight is, what gives the author a sense of achievement and satisfaction, what justifies the expenditure of time, energy, initiative—what the author's *interest* is—one might be forgiven for thinking it is spirit. "Theism" and "theological" are used almost interchangeably for the presence of spirit, and spirit in turn appears in the words "animism" and "vitalism."

François Jacob's *The Logic of Life,* its epigraph looking to the overthrow of "all the schools of theology, all the churches of the earth," is a history of the development of modern biology. The ultimate vision is of a system that is utterly without purpose or direction, and in which the words "higher" and "lower" have no place. But this vision has one continuous and striking exception, which is the evolution of biology itself, over centuries, working itself pure of any element of "vitalism." The contrast between Jacob's all-encompassing account of the biological, which, like Changeux's, must include the phenomenon of biology itself, and Jacob's account of the evolution of this all-encompassing account of the biological, in which he himself participated, fairly leaps from the page. Jacob's pressing ahead despite the contrast points to motivation and back to the epigraph. It raises the question whether "all the churches of the world" might not be necessary to the science that evokes antiscience.

In the exchange between neurobiologist Changeux and mathematician Alain Connes in their *Conversations* on mind and matter, "faith," like "belief," becomes a negative term. The biologist refers to "your vehement profession of faith—because you admit that's what it is" (p. 44), and observes that "belief in the existence of a mathematical truth outside the human mind requires an act of faith that the majority of formalist-minded mathematicians are not aware of making." (p. 42) Only once does the mathematician respond to this confidence so evidently based upon axiom, and without the support of the direct experience the mathematician himself was reporting.

"How can you be so sure?" (p. 50) he says. That the mathematician does *not* say, "But yours is only a faith," or, less civilly, "You seem no different from a fundamentalist thumping his book," or say anything like it, but only the mild "How can you be so sure?" is perhaps attributable to his own tie to the position from which the biologist is speaking. We have noted it before—an exception only for mathematics is in issue in this conversation between them, at least on the surface, and the mathematician too has his total theory that would make pleading for an exception unnecessary. What he cannot bring himself to call "mere faith," even when he is being accused of "mere faith," may have as its content and perhaps its defining content an animus like Changeux's toward theism, purpose, spirit.

Recall the "savage thought" of which the physicist Roger Penrose is presented as an example. It is a savage thought that "would amount to assigning specifically human qualities to external reality." (p. 200) That this is Emerson's thought, the thought Lewis Thomas strains toward in *The Fragile Species,* the thought anyone entertains who wants to avoid any radical separation of the human and human experience from nature and experience of nature, is no bar to its contemptuous dismissal as "savage." A more recent argument written for popular consumption, William Calvin's *How Brains Think: Evolving Intelligence, Then and Now,*[2] read and reviewed as a "fine," "exhilarating," and "inspiring" rebuttal of Penrose,[3] concludes that "consciousness physicists" use "mathematical concepts to dazzle rather than enlighten. . . . [S]uch theorists usually avoid the word 'spirit' and say something about quantum fields." What triggers—or animates—both response and delight in the response is sense of spirit.

Within mathematics itself, one of the recent works in the continuing debate over the nature of mathematics is Brian Rotman's *Ad Infinitum.*[4] The debate is especially between so-called constructivists, whom the biologist Changeux adopted as his own, and so-called realists, believing in an ultimate mathematical reality, with whom the mathematician Connes identifies. *Ad Infinitum* focuses on the meaning and use of infinity in mathematical and scientific thought. It is full of interest, sensitive in new ways to the place of language and person in mathematical and scientific thought. But *Ad Infinitum* is not an exploration and a questioning. It is a spirited attack, with its strongest language, the most cutting, the most damning, incorporating some reference to theism.

Rotman begins with the divine, and ends with it. What he has said in between is fertile and provocative. But it is the "unstated theism—implicit and unacknowledged—of twentieth-century mathematical infinitism" (p. 157) that is his ultimate refutation of mathematicians who use infinity. He assumes the persuasive force, for his intended audience, of his characterization of his mathematical opponents, recalling the refrain of "no one" in Changeux and Connes's exchange ("no one" could think this, "no one" would think that), or the picture of Searle saying the same while standing among the Hindus. In his case, like others speaking of spirit, the drumbeat of reference to God and the divine is such that we may wonder not only why there has been such concern with the divine, such lifelong motivation focused upon the divine. We may wonder how the divine could be spoken of without a sense of what it is that is being spoken of—how one so focused can avoid being betrayed by the very use of the word.

THE CONNECTION BETWEEN MOTIVE AND CONTENT

Motive and content, motive blending into content where these largest of matters are concerned: any of us might pursue this *prima facie* case with a larger survey, and a closer and more attentive reading of language which is common enough now to lose its power to shock, and to pass without notice. Much the same is being done in modern scholarship on that great negative of the twentieth century, anti-Semitism: larger surveys, closer and more attentive reading of language that tended to pass without notice because it was so common. It marks also modern attempts to define, understand, and trace the implications of racism in the United States before and after slavery, the changing place of women and the feminine in the eighteenth and nineteenth centuries.

The thought then might beckon, after larger survey and closer reading, that "science" is defined in essence and in detail, is molded by and is inseparable from the enemy it constructs to hate. Noticeable ugliness would then be intrinsic, that ugliness which is to be seen in the late twentieth century, which has for many a particular look of its own and is beyond and quite different from any mere robust openness in dispute.

"Read what is actually said, look at it," says the feminist, the person of color writing history or arguing policy. So here. Notice what is said, it might be urged, even as the anti-Semitic is now noticed. As that great negative, which successfully reduced selected human beings to vermin in the first half of the twentieth century, might have next set its sights on others selected by their denial of its all-encompassing premises,[5] this negative too has a wide compass. Recall Searle and the Hindus who had not heard the news, Weinberg and his anticipated war with Islam after the battle with the Christians, Changeux's characterization of all religious and ethical belief as "infection" like a "viral attack." (p. 227) Suppose, given the breadth of this negative, that the line between the child and the song sparrow really is threatened: Go to the Holocaust Memorial Museum and lean over the wall that protects the unsuspecting from sudden encounter with the monitors running the captured photographs, and look at the children in the research laboratories, the man being gradually crushed by air pressure.[6] Or look again at the films taken from the University of Pennsylvania of bound primates being subjected to head trauma. Whatever you think of its medical justification, listen to the mocking that accompanies the smashing.[7] Meanness and smallness spread. Hatred feeds and is fed.

THE ROUND OF NEGATION AND THE PECULIAR PROBLEM OF HUMAN CONNECTION

Why is there this ugliness, this contempt so open toward so many, billions indeed, each on his or her own journey in the cosmos? Dickens sketched ugliness whenever he heard nineteenth-century industrial capitalism being presented as a total system. Why this association?

Why is there ever ugliness? Destructiveness and self-destructiveness are variously explained. Recognizable patterns of adolescent psychology do fit aspects of late-twentieth-century cosmological speculation. It does not reach too far for human universals to see something similar, the psychology of the adolescent who doesn't understand, and who destroys—torn by the prospect of responsibility, attracted to the undifferentiated mass—in the teenage armies of China's Cultural Revolution, another of the twentieth century's experiments with the total. A professed view of human language and meaning in language that would eliminate both human language and meaning is common. It is essential, for instance, to apocalyptic visions of construction of superhuman intelligences that will inevitably eliminate the merely human in evolutionary competition— dates are set for this final destruction.[8] In reflecting on what he has seen in his time of those driven by such visions, Joseph Weizenbaum comments, "I think it fundamentally has to do with power, and certainly with the power to make life." He goes on, in explanation, to wonder whether an unacknowledged envy by men of women's capacity to "give birth to new life"[9] may play a part.

But explanation has its own pitfalls. The question "why?" can be asked even about the asking: why do we, or you, or I ask "why"? Think of any one of us saying, offering, asserting something. The saying, offering, asserting invites our doing and saying something ourselves. The saying or asserting that hits our ears may be addressed to the wind or ocean, and we can pass by and not disturb the speaker; but if it is addressed to us, it is an invitation. And when it is an *explanation* that is offered and pressed, we can respond by engaging in *explanation* ourselves, imitate, as it were—we can stay in the world of explanation, within the form that world takes.

The totalitarian social and political theories that lay behind the Holocaust and Gulag and other of the special experiences of the twentieth century were, after all, theories of explanation. The prison interrogations in Arthur Koestler's mid-century *Darkness at Noon*[10] were mandatory discussions of what must be the predictable consequence of dialectical materialism, a total vision of structure and— all else—superstructure, embraced, it was thought, on both sides of the interrogation table. The deep intertwining of the political and the explanatory in the total vision of fascism may be recalled again. It can be glimpsed in the presentation to the faculty of the Reich University of Strasbourg at its first plenary meeting in 1942: "The pair of terms 'organism and environment,' the topic of this evening, means nothing other in the language of biology than the phrase 'blood and soil' in the language of politics."[11]

With those theories of explanation Elias Canetti struggled heroically. Scientifically trained, German, European, novelist and theorist both, he was caught by them and haunted by them, wanting to understand them and insisting on *explaining* those explanations that were total. Finally in *Crowds and Power* (1960)[12] Canetti, who was eventually to receive a Nobel Prize (in literature) like many we are reading here, pursued a total theory equally dark and ultimately destructive that did not exempt himself.

Such response in kind, explanation of explanation, which if it could be truly closed would be the end, can most certainly proceed from an unwillingness to separate oneself as a human being from the human beings one analyzes and addresses. If others are torturers or destroyers, even self-destroyers, and they are not different, then it must be accepted that one is oneself a destroyer and self-destroyer; and this is a position that can be based as much on modesty, or on a sense of innate and intrinsic connection despite individuality, as on any direct sense of one's own inclinations and capacities in this regard. There is this dilemma in human connection.

We have noted the dilemma before and will come to it again. The assumption on the part of others speaking to us that we are like them, and our assumption listening to them that they are like us, can work two ways. What we know they must know also. What we must assume, what our actions and words reveal to us who do and speak them, they must assume also, and their actions and words reveal to them. And reveal to us.

But now let us think that moving through this dilemma might be what candor offers, especially at this point in the unrolling of thought when it seems most needed. The Elias Canetti who includes himself in the frenzy of crowds and the grasp for power is also the Canetti with the capacity for such deep shock at the Holocaust that he wrote *Crowds and Power*. He is the Canetti who obviously found worth in writing *Crowds and Power* and in addressing it to us all, rather than falling into silence, or dying. There are affirmations implicit in his bothering. In his very attempt to persuade there are affirmations. And, given the two directions connection runs, the one who destroys and self-destroys in social and political life may also be like *this* Canetti.

That this is so would counsel against taking the route represented by Canetti's *Crowds and Power,* theory swallowing theory. Any of us can dissent from Canetti, and begin the journey of explaining his explanation. Certainly the route is open toward something similar to *Crowds and Power,* where the new totalism in the second half of the twentieth century is in cosmological vision rather than in social or political theory. The pursuit of explanation of the explainer, and with the explainer the explainer's explanation of himself and us, is always possible. But we may view the ever-present possibility of it as an argument against total theory as such, our own total theory, or another's. We can forgo taking yet one more step along the road that is littered with explanations that explain oneself as they explain others. We can stop, and listen to each other instead.

REVOLUTIONARY NEGATION

We must look, before continuing, at one more aspect of the negative familiar in the twentieth century. Associated with the route of explaining the explainer, rather than listening and asking for candor, is another response that purports to forgo any theory whatever, and with it the persuasion of minds that any theory involves, in favor of direct action. If the negative is what pushes and molds construction and elaboration of models, if the negative is the source of interest, is the initiative for work and the drive behind resourcefulness and tenacity in argument, if the imagination is feeding on the negative, then the argument (it may be said) is not one to respond to as argument, or even to try to understand.

Evil is never understood. For some—the Hitlers, the Stalins, the Pol Pots—the human connection may have to be severed. Evil resists either explanation or sympathetic understanding—full evil does, if our talk of evil wishes to introduce degrees of it (rather than call anything that is less than evil a relative degree of wrong). The very perception of evil is the urge to destroy it—perception and reaction are one and the same.

Here, though it be allowed that what is being said and urged and done is on this side of evil (if that is allowed), the object would be *change*. Negative evokes negative. The consequences of change may not be perceptible much beyond destruction. But there is often seen a faith implicit or sometimes explicit that, just as imagination can give the unpredicted and unpredictable, so providence working with a clean slate will provide a positive that cannot be described in advance; or the nature of human nature, benign when no longer distorted, will provide a new positive.

This, the revolutionary response, is familiar enough to us now. There is a strain of it in the Christianity of the Gospels, if not in the Christianity of tradition. It is the prophetic side of Marxism,[13] addressed to the cold systems of market capitalism, and not all the economic and medical and agricultural gains in the world are enough to strike a bargain, any more than they were for Pol Pot as he was going about changing Cambodia to its very roots. Revolutionary responses of this kind can be seen in radical feminism, and in the "radical critique" of liberal society that occupies various schools and that appears in the study of the phenomenon of law under various names.

And among the responses that Lewis Thomas would describe as "antiscience" are some that do go far beyond the renewed interest in magic among the educated that he noted, and far beyond a loss of interest in supporting research with public funds or a failure of transmission of scientific work and habits in education. They call for total change and may have no compunctions, despite the experience of the twentieth century, at using force to achieve it.

READING THE WHOLE EVIDENCE

But negative need not beget negative. Response need not take the form of that which calls forth response. A sense of science, or of the scientist, is not to be determined on only part of the evidence. Science is a human endeavor, engaged in by human beings. What is said, within particular fields of science and social science, or about the nature of science as such, or about the nature of the human world that includes science or the world that includes the human world, is said by human beings, and not in unison, but one to one and one by one. Each is on his journey through life, his only journey (perhaps his only journey, if we put aside what billions say to the Westerner venturing to the other half of the globe). To any but those who say they believe the world is illusion, or a creation and emanation solely of the human imagination, to any who acknowledge incarnate being and—as they face their situation in the cosmos— acknowledge a material constitution that is not peculiar to themselves, science brings gifts, of fascination, of beauty, of relief from pain, gifts of unclouded thought, of freedom to love; and in fact these gifts and their effects are enjoyed even by those who live in a world whose material constitution they deny.

Of the likenesses in twentieth-century social and political thought that total theory of the cosmological kind calls to mind one, we might think, is racism. Not just the racism boiling beneath the Second World War and offering to define all who lived in the world: A reader who has lived through racial discrimination in the United States can resonate to the "all" in the proposition "race is all." But the particularities of race, at least in the southern United States in the twentieth century, may be beyond theory; personal love and imitation may be too intertwined with personal humiliation and personal cruelty. Between men and women relations are complex beyond theory, respect and exploitation side by side and emerging not from different directions but from the same person. It is this very sameness of source that allows appeals to be made—appeals, rather than war and destruction—to the person who is yet beyond the person from whom both respect and exploitation come.

So it is with those who identify themselves as "scientists" or "mathematicians." The negative when it is in them is not in them all by itself. "The materialist program" we can recall the neurobiologist Changeux explaining to the mathematician Connes is "an act of self-discipline" by which one tries to "eliminate" in oneself "all remaining traces of transcendence." (p. 25) This program, this discipline of the self, does not just happen, unless one disregards Changeux's own description of it and extrapolates—not following Changeux but on one's own, because it would be one's own extrapolation, not one Changeux makes back to himself: *his* words, with regard to himself, are words of purpose, of trying. There is choice in this drive, but there is not just "choice"—a system, a machine, a switch, can "choose": there is desire, will, action, initiative, attention, rousing of the mind, imagination.

One cannot understand Changeux's "materialist program" at all, the negative drive, the thirst for elimination ("all traces"), if one adopts Changeux's total theory in which all merely happens. One would not do that even on Changeux's account, unless one read only part of what Changeux was saying and not, as any lawyer would urge you to do, the whole. It is hard in fact really to read only part and not the whole. The Legionnaires of the Archangel Michael in Romania during the 1940s swore oaths of obedience, drank each others' blood, and put packets of Romanian soil around their necks, so that the eyes of the children whom they rounded up would mean no more to them than the eyes of sparrows that they netted. The juxtaposition with total theory in science or mathematics may seem cruel, but they too were engaged in an act of self-discipline seeking to eliminate the humanity within them and the linked perception of humanity in others.[14] But because in either case it *is* a drive, a program, and does not just happen within like a mad rage erupts in the violent insane, the person sits in judgment on it, and so do others sit in judgment on it.

There are drives, programs, visions in addition to this one, even where the "materialist program" is found. Fascination, beauty, clarity, freedom are there too. So, when Changeux or any other argues and appeals to any of us, or, like Changeux with Connes, to one who is identified as one of their own, the reach is not merely for the negative (drumbeat though the negative is, when discussion and argument are replayed and listened to). When someone seeks to be listened to, and seeks to augment his voice by identifying himself as "scientist," and to situate himself among scientists, it is not the negative that one uses to identify him as a scientist. It is not, in general, negation that evokes from us a turn to listen to a voice.

At the end of Steven Weinberg's *Dreams of a Final Theory*, in which he expresses surprise that "even from scientists" one hears "occasional hints of vitalism, the belief in biological processes that cannot be explained in terms of physics and chemistry" (p. 246), he recounts interviews with a number of cosmologists and physicists who were asked what they thought of his remark at the end of his widely used short 1977 book *The First Three Minutes,* "The more the universe seems comprehensible, the more it also seems pointless." Weinberg was interested in numbers, majorities and minorities, agreements and disagreements. Ten agreed and thirteen did not, but of those thirteen who disagreed, he noted, three disagreed because they did not see why anyone would *expect* to find such a thing as purpose.

The question the ordinary juror called up to listen to this might then be expected to ask, ask of the "scientist," is "Why do you care?— How can you care, about anything?" But the question is rarely asked or pressed, because the "scientist" evidently does care. The economist who introduces the device of economic man, the wholly self-aggrandizing profit maximizer, to explore the workings of the systems of our own making in which we find ourselves—for we know we are situated in systems monetary, productive, and distributive, and that we do not understand them—slips from presupposition to apparent belief and asserts that man is economic man and only economic man. His friends might be expected to shrink away, his children to glance over their shoulder at him, his doctors to become concerned, the local prosecutor to become alert. But they do not.

Chapter Six

THE FUNDAMENTAL ACKNOWLEDGMENT IN SCIENTIFIC THOUGHT

Science and fear of science: can we say science as such is characterized by the totalitarian in its ultimate view, and the scientist identified by belief in it? I do not think we can. Moreover I think candor with one another will eventually lead to agreement that we cannot say this. Candor will not do all. It does not and will not lead to agreement on all things, or joint understanding of all things. But in the largest matters it may lead, by itself as it were, to joint understanding. In the largest matters it may go further than in smaller matters.

Before our skirting just now the temptation to negation, and when we were initially considering the question of identifying science and scientist, we noted the fact of assent, both the phenomenon and the necessity of it. It is common, all around us—we do not go too far calling it a fact. It is this necessary fact of assent that bridges any gulf of vision between science and what is not science, and that keeps "he who is not with me is against me" from attending the very perception of their difference. In its light, the one is not the negative of the other.

PERSUASION WITHIN AND BEYOND
THE SCIENTIFIC WORLD

Let us remember again that neither the scientist—neurobiologist, chemist, physicist—nor the mathematician, who is sometimes called "scientist," can let truth take care of itself. Scientists and mathematicians do not let truth take care of itself. They need to persuade, as they need air to live.

They need assent from others on matters particular to their field: assent among scientists, within science. They also need assent within their field on any vision of the nature of things that includes their field and themselves and includes others who are outside the field and outside the group they would call "themselves": visions that they would put to the rest of the world.

Then, they need assent from that "rest of the world"—or some substantial enough or valued part of it—on the visions they would put forth of the nature of the rest of the world. They need to persuade *us,* just as "they" need to persuade each other. I should think the need to persuade us is a reason for the drumbeat of mutual attack that can be heard *within* science and the readiness to attack that is reflected in Lewis Thomas's confessions and avoidances.

"They" need assent not for the continuing transfer of food and leisure to them that makes possible their work. They need assent because without assent they themselves do not have proof of their vision. Each failure of persuasion is a brick taken from the foundations of their own thought about the world. Law and lawyers have long experience with this: it is part of the recurring basis for torture to secure confessions, for without the assent of the accused, in the face of vigorous and authentic dissent, doubt remains and doubt grows. There may be some instances, the Eureka! of individual mathematical illumination being one of them, that no amount of dissent or failure to persuade could shake. There are lonely faiths. But with regard to the nature of a world which is not entirely an emanation from oneself or one's own creation, it may not be possible even to think, to think or to conceive what one proposes to think, without assent or the prospect of assent beyond.

AUTHENTICITY AND ACKNOWLEDGMENT

The necessity of assent to a view of the world produces the possibility of dissent. It may be authentic dissent, or it may not—it may be strategic. Authenticity is a matter for one to judge who faces dissent to a vision he or she has proffered, and also for one looking on the situation from the outside to judge. But that is just as much the case where assent appears. To one looking on the situation from outside, and to one seeking assent, there is no assent, with the assurance it provides, if it is not authentic assent. Assent by bribe, by drugs, by torture, under hallucination, determined in any way by factors that have nothing to do with the appeal of the vision itself, does not serve, and, depending on our understanding of what is embraced by "causation," this can be true of any assent causally determined, perceptibly causally determined—in the perception of either one looking on outside, or of one appealing for assent.

That there can be authentic assent and authentic dissent, the legally trained tend somewhat naturally to see. In the humanities as well as the social sciences, indeed within churches, it is very easy to slip into the fixation "I am right, the other is wrong," and thence into attack not greatly different from the attack associated with total theories of a cosmological kind or with totalitarianism in politics. But it does no good for one without power of purse or sword to keep saying "I am right," for that one is, after all, only one. There are others, also speaking.

This the lawyer is trained to see without concluding because of it—the fact a speaker is only one and there are other speakers—that truth must be only the outcome of a process, a resolution of forces. Unlike others who can be heard saying they see any and every human conclusion as no more than a cultural artifact which is the product of continuously changing social and political forces, the lawyer must act, as well as listen and comment, and act in situations in which he or she must also secure assent; and the lawyer must then live with responsibility for the infliction of terrible pains and disappointments. In neither, securing the assent of others nor living with responsibility for consequences of action, could he or she be sustained, as person, or in identity as lawyer and decision-maker, by a vision in which there was nothing but outcomes of processes, resolutions of forces.

Imagine you are in a lonely cabin in the dusk. Is that a wolf rather than a ram outside the cabin, moving slowly, indistinct? Others are with you. There is dissension. There is action to take or not to take, with consequences attending either course. To the lawyer in you the important aspect of the situation is not that the proposition "wolf," "ram," is empirically verifiable, in theory, which might be the important aspect for the scientist in you. To the lawyer the important aspect of the situation is the authenticity, the credibility, of those who are speaking toward one view or another. To the lawyer, indeed, empirical verification itself would present questions of testimony, if a scout were sent out and came back to speak, or if the scout did not return. And it is no help to action to abandon both the empirical and the authentic and say (as is said) that whether there is a wolf outside is only the product of a process inside the cabin, which will work its way the way it does, or that the testimony and positions of those arguing toward assent or moving toward dissent are discountable not just for various reasons and to various degrees, but ultimately entirely discountable as the product of forces operating, in which authenticity and responsibility have no place.

The lawyer knows that a speaker is only one and that there are other speakers, but does not assume that the speaker's words are no access to truth because no one's could be, or move to numerical methods of resolution without inquiring who is speaking and what her reasons are (whether the question is the existence of a wolf, or the existence of the law, or the existence of a criminal mind in the accused). But then, neither does the scientist. Nor the mathematician. They—we, if we can call ourselves scientists or mathematicians— do not believe that the world they describe or their description of it is a collective fiction. They may not have to take action in the way a lawyer does, except in the allocation of salaries, research funds, or access to the public forum of publication, but they thirst to reach a conclusion of which they are assured.

If there is dissent, they must face it, and not simply treat it like a blackball in a vote to be put on one side of a box. Even if they were not constrained by the law of murder, they know it would do them no good to simply destroy dissent. If they did succeed in killing the dissenter so that he or she was no more in the material world with them, that would not mean for them there was therefore no dissent.

In *facing* dissent, scientist and mathematician must seek to persuade, and not simply manipulate a process. If they thought one whose assent they sought was simply a process to be manipulated toward an outcome, they would not bother. The outcome would not help them toward what they seek, which is what to know or believe themselves. If they thought *all* others were processes to be manipulated, they would be alone in the world, and must wonder not only why they cared to ask their questions but how they could ever be assured the answers that come to mind were not mistaken or foolish. And if they thought they themselves were only processes being manipulated, they would not be asking the questions or thirsting for answers.

In *facing* dissent, scientists and mathematicians look to the person of the dissenter, to the authenticity of the dissenter's position, to competence, to reasons, and to credibility: by which we mean believability which in turn implies the possibility of belief both on the part of the one who is believable and on the part of the one who perceives the belief.

THE CONSEQUENCE OF DISSENT

Believability and belief and what is believed—we cannot really disentangle what is believed from whether it is believed, or, in the end, from the believer.

If, confronted now with efforts to persuade, counterarguments, further evidence, the dissenter continues to dissent and says he is not persuaded, that is not the end of the matter. The dissenter does not have to agree. There is no "have to" where there is a question and the question is a vision of things. The one persuading must make a decision, about the authenticity of the disagreement or contrary vision; but that decision cannot be made by simply examining whether, "objectively" in some sense, the contrary vision is different from his own vision.

First he must determine what the disagreement is about, what the contrary position is and how his own position is being read. To do this, he must translate between persons and acknowledge the possible difference in their languages—to translate, he must acknowledge another person, and acknowledge that his own language is not the only language in the world. Then he inquires into the good faith, the motivation, the competence, the experience of the one dissenting, and in doing that (which he has done in translating also) he acknowledges another person who is capable of sincerity, belief, and judgment.

If the other still says "I do not agree" despite more argument and new evidence, and the persuader remains convinced of the other's sincerity and competence and confident of his own translation, he can only rethink his own position or continue in the effort to persuade. Of course he can rethink his conclusion about the authenticity or competence of the dissenter; but as to that, he must monitor himself carefully and ask himself whether *he* is being authentic in his own conclusion about the authenticity or competence of the other. Each time he dismisses another whom he actually thinks to be authentic or competent, he undermines his own assurance.

If, finally, the persuader or proposer *must* choose, between himself and those who agree with him on the one hand, and, on the other, those who disagree with him whose disagreement he cannot shake nor yet dismiss as merely the product of ignorance or bad faith or the product of forces beyond the dissenter's control, *then he must choose by entering belief*: belief in his perception of a truth which is not a truth emerging from statistical or numerical operations according to rules, since those very "rules" are in question. In his choosing he acknowledges a substance that is not patterned process perceptible simply as pattern. He has moved from the individual, and from process, to something that is beyond the individual, and beyond process.

There need be no explicit claim to authority—in scientific usage the word "authority" is a pejorative, the pejorative opposite of the demonstrated. But the reach for the sanction of science, and the search within oneself for the voice of the scientist or of the mathematician, is a reach for an identity just as in the phenomenon of human authority generally. There is an appeal to an identity that matches the identity of an individual in its irreducibility, an identity in which the individual participates and which lives, even if it lives only through one individual. The reach and appeal is for the same effect as is seen and experienced in the phenomenon of human authority generally: focused attention among the billions of possible voices—a voice augmented—and deference (which is a form of assent) through internalization of voice and joinder ultimately of individual with individual.

At every point in living with the necessity of assent, and with the flow of implications of the necessity of assent in a world in which there are many of us, there is acknowledgment of the person, the reality of the person: the person as judge, the person who believes and whose assent is valuable, the person who does not believe and whose nonbelief is troubling.

It is this fundamental acknowledgment that makes it impossible to say that "science," invoked and attracting attention to and augmenting the voice of an individual passing through adult life, is the negative or is total theory or one of the total theories urged—or that "antiscience" should itself be an eliminative and eradicating project. Belief about the nature of the world can be yearned for and worked toward, with argument about it, contention and strong urgings. But at some level, in some way, there is always recognition of an openness about it, this nature of the world that we are drawn to discuss and express as if by spell cast on us, openness we ourselves introduce, and represent.

Chapter Seven

WAYS OF KNOWING AND THE QUESTION OF SCIENTIFIC METHOD

What we have been discussing is in the substance of scientific thought. Let us turn to scientific method.

THE DISTINCTIVENESS OF SCIENTIFIC METHOD

We all engage in scientific method, whether or not we are identified as scientists, and we have been taught that scientific method is distinctive. It may be thought that the fundamental acknowledgment of the person, and of the necessity of assent as a given of the world as it really is, transgresses a line of difference, a gulf indeed, extending at least as far back as Bacon. The one side of this gulf is method that looks to texts and the voices of others. I have called this, for mnemonic purposes, the legal form of thought, though it is an ordinary and daily manner of proceeding in human life. The other side of this gulf is method that looks to experimental results, to confirmation and verification that cannot be denied without insanity or deficit in the physical senses.

But there is not such a line of difference or gulf between methods as might be thought, quite aside from the first and obvious necessity of determining (of course by human decision, with assent) whether there is insanity or what constitutes a deficit in the senses when there is a line of difference between individuals. And, insofar as purity in the practice of scientific method is associated with a separable identity of an individual as "a scientist," there may not be such a difference, by this measure, between scientists and nonscientists as might be thought.

It is obviously important that what is called the scientific form of thought, contrasted with the legal form of thought, be defended, maintained, and taught. Much that is positive in the modern world, the source of our satisfaction in living now and our skepticism about even our own nostalgia for an earlier age, flows from work focused by the presuppositions of scientific work. Much in the maintenance of the human enterprise of science depends upon the disciplining effect of an offer of and a presumption of ultimate verifiability without regard to person. Look, see, try it yourself, don't take my word for it, we do not have to agree, we do not have to depend on one another or defer to one another—we are citizens in the ultimate democracy of fact.

But in the world and in fact, scientific method, powerful, liberating, and disciplining though it is, operates only in the context of and in utter dependence on methods it contrasts itself to. Not merely law and the method that gives us law. The human experience of time and the human experience of individual death are alone enough to situate scientific method within more general ways of proceeding.

Science, its methods and its conclusions, must be taught and continuously taught to generations seamlessly succeeding one another. No individual and no generation can verify all for itself, see, touch all, by itself. We may suppose there is a running test of what has come before, in each new experiment that builds on it, confirmation and disconfirmation all quite automatic. When someone builds on teaching that cannot be demonstrated to him in his lifetime and suddenly finds himself confounded or surprised, has he not tested underpinnings and found them wanting? Is he not rerunning history and seeing for himself? But all may be in true: surprise may be the beginning of a basic movement in thought, a perception of something new about the world. Surprise may be a high point of a life in science, not at all a dismantling or step back. And should defect be the source of surprise, there is no finger which points to a particular part of the scaffolding that is not in true. Time is running, the builder must turn to others. But another's report of a weakness found will be just that, a report, asking for credence.

All are dependent upon good faith in reports of past results and confirmation of past results, good faith in preserving the archive which does not stay with us by itself, good faith in reports of new results and confirmation of new results. All are dependent upon choices made in the continuous teaching, the teachers themselves dependent as much as students. These dependencies depend upon person, acknowledge person, and what the introduction of person into the world of experience introduces in turn—substance and depth, dignity, respect.

Mathematics is not exempt, even mathematics in the form called pure where method blends with direct perception or illumination. "There is no mathematician so pure that he feels no interest at all in the physical world; but, in so far as he succumbs to this temptation, he will be abandoning his purely mathematical position," the mathematician G. H. Hardy observed in *A Mathematician's Apology*. There is a mathematical world to be inhabited, as there is a world of scientific achievement. "Realists" among mathematicians (as their school is called), such as G. H. Hardy or Alain Connes whom we have heard here, who perceive and believe in their perception of a transcendent mathematical reality, often present a complete picture. "You conceive of my external mathematical reality as a part of the external physical world," replies Connes to the neurobiologist Changeux seeking to persuade him to the neurobiologist's own complete picture. "For me, it's just the opposite: external physical reality is a part of archaic mathematical reality." (*Conversations*, p. 206) G. H. Hardy had said before that the most important difference between mathematician and physicist "seems to me to be this, that the mathematician is in much more direct contact with reality."[1]

But even the nonmathematician can observe that assurance of this cosmology is not a matter of direct contact, however much the experience of archaic mathematical reality may be. The confidence that drives the urging of its completeness, the satisfaction in its totality, rests upon a sense of mathematics as a whole that allows mathematicians to think of "it" as a world and reality; and that sense in turn rests upon the testimony of others working in the various branches of mathematics, no matter how fine and comprehensive a mathematician may be at the peak of his powers and fullness of his learning. With dependence on testimony come the presuppositions and implications of believing—internalizing—the statements and beliefs of others.

There is nothing abject about this dependence. There is action and responsibility in choosing what to reject and what to weigh. There is nothing automatic about it, nothing absolutely required, nothing of an authoritarian cast. Decision is personal, as is deciding what is sufficient—in the face of dissent—to satisfy and fortify to the point of belief. Connections to the fundamental acknowledgment we touched upon in the last chapter are evident. With regard to how conclusions are reached, particularly about ultimate reality or the nature of the world, the methods of mathematics are not purely mathematical. For "realist" mathematicians, the purely mathematical world may be beyond the physical world, the physical world a reflection of the mathematical reality. It is not beyond the person, person listening, or person heard.

THE WHATNESS OF THE VERIFIABLE

Returning to the reality that is offered by scientific verification, we can see these same dependencies in the determination of *what* it is that is being verified. That must rest upon translation between human languages of which there are many and perhaps as many as there are individual human beings.

Results in physics are, perhaps, only occasionally subject to such open-endedness if they merge with and are expressed through the devices of mathematics—it is the very limitation to what is said to be "precisely defined" which characterizes an object as "a mathematical object" or admits a subject of discussion into a mathematics department of a university.

But when experimental method is extended to matters of general human experience, the question of *what* is being proven or confirmed is constant, and the passage of time, the continuous inexorable passage of time, ensures that a question of translation is constant in the reading of past results and confirmations. Look, see, try it yourself: the question is the "it."

We can any of us run experiments on love, on music, on language, on law, on authority, on sense of self (assuming, we should say, that experiments on love are possible without killing it). But the results are subject to judgment by others that it *is* love, language, music, law, authority, or sense of self with which we have been experimenting, and the addition of careful specification, elaborateness of protocol, and trained investigators does not make the results any less subject to such judgment. Where total theory is in question, extending as it does forward into all and everything human, this condition is always present, this limitation on the difference experimental method introduces and on the distinctiveness of experimental method.

THE OBVIOUS LIMITS ON VERIFICATION

Then, too, where human matters are concerned there are experiments that cannot be verified and results that cannot be repeated, so long at least as the line between song sparrow and child is kept. If the question is how auditory and musical capacities are associated with the development of neural systems in the song sparrow, the sparrow is deafened, or separated from parents, or killed so that its brain can be sliced and stained. If the same question is raised about the auditory and musical capacities of the child, we or anyone must currently wait for experiments to present themselves by chance: a deaf child, not a child that has been deafened; a child that happens to have been locked away, not a child who is experimentally locked away; a child who dies, not a child who is killed; a child who dies as to whom adequate permission can be obtained to slice and stain her brain.

To have it said, "We know the human body can consume itself beyond its fatty parts and continue to live for an extended time," and, to the question properly posed by experimental method—"What is the source of that, how might that be verified, confirmed by repetition?"— have the reply "We know that from Auschwitz," there comes a pause, currently, so long as it is not in fact believed that man is "just a system" like a leaf, or, perhaps, a song sparrow. Repetition is not the next step. The next step may be the reverse of repetition: The Environmental Protection Agency in the United States, commissioning a study on the effect on human beings of phosgene gas, ordered that data on human exposure from experiments in concentration camps be excluded—though to the experimenters there, according to what they seemed to say in part of what they said as a whole, there was no line between their subjects and animal subjects in other experiments.[2]

And, of course, where experiment must wait, and must depend on small numbers, or even a single individual, the assumption of likeness between human individuals comes under particularly heavy pressure. The assumption more evidently relies upon the phenomenon— the experience—of the person, the identity sensed one with another despite physical difference, the left-handed with the right-handed, the gifted with the nongifted, the normal with the Down's syndrome child.

THE CONSEQUENCE OF HUMAN INDIVIDUATION

This leads to an addendum to any method of actual repeatable observation. Not quite a limitation on it, and beyond its dependence, there can be seen a supplementing of it which blends it with other ways to belief. We canvassed this without particular reference to method in the last chapter and should touch on it further here, because method has so strong a call.

Despite what may be said by any of us, each of us is an expert on himself. Each of us is on his own journey through the cosmos. At times one may think that one's own is the only journey there is. Each of us is in a position to deny what is said about us, or a vision of the world that includes us. The other, the person speaking, is but one, and on a journey which for him or her may be the only journey. "I" (or "you") am also at least one, and on a journey: the world is yours and mine, as much as it is the speaker's own.

Insofar as the speaker's proposition about the world reaches us (as all total theory seeks to do, including not just the speaker but us and all we know and experience), we are fully, fully, in command, cosmologically in command as it were. This is in the very nature of our individual separation. If someone else undertakes to demonstrate to you that you are wrong about yourself, the appeal is still to you as judge.

"You are absolute goodness," it may be said. "No, I am not," we may think or say, with more or less full confidence, and we may go on to wonder whether the other means it, or, rather, what is almost the same, go on to wonder *what* the other means. "You are evil," it may be said. Equally can we say, "No, I am not," and say this also with some confidence—the lawyer knows this well and sees something like this said regularly, whenever the convict continues to protest his innocence, and the lawyer must face the epistemological dilemma in knowing we can say something confidently about ourselves against the conclusions of others. Any proposition to us about ourselves we are in a position utterly to deny—it being always remembered that what the proposition is, if we grant the other is like ourselves, remains always a live question and that words, the words of the proposition, do not define themselves.

Someone saying, quite to the contrary, that we have no knowledge of ourselves, we only act—as the ant acts[3]—and are to be read in those actions, which are as open to be read by someone else as by us, is only making a proposition about us. There is some attraction in it insofar as we can understand it, for our actions do tell us things about ourselves and we do read ourselves as a whole, our actions as well as our words and glances, all our actions and all our words and glances together. But insofar as we take it as a proposition to us that we know nothing that the other doesn't know, we can deny it. "There is something inside us you have not taken account of," we can say. The gifted mathematician says this every time he proposes an insight, and others around can say they do not see it, and it is nothing, but the mathematician will not agree—unless the perception of those around him is important to his own perception.

Of course if someone says, not about us but about herself, "Deep inside me there are jewels," then adds, "You are like me," many of us would likely say, "*No,* I am flesh and blood." But that would only emphasize for us that the other can equally say this "No" to what we might propose. Someone might similarly appeal to likeness out of concern for you (for *you,* as an individual), not imperiously, might argue to you for instance that you are best off taking a drug because you are like the human subjects on which the drug was experimentally tested. You can still say that you are different. Anyone can dismiss what you say as mad, or without evidence, and convince himself on the basis of the evidence he has, and general assumption. But he cannot convince himself by experiment and particular observation: cannot, that is, so long as he has concern for you and sees you as an individual, so long as the line between the child and the sparrow does not fade and you are not put in the same place as the sparrow.

To be sure, human beings might think they have no such concern, as we have seen. Someone saying there is nothing really "inside" us, or nothing of the sort to which one or another of us may be referring, could contemplate killing us if we resist to the death, opening us up, and looking for himself as his method instructs him to do. If he did, it might not matter to him that we would be gone and beyond persuasion on the evidence he sees. But after satisfying himself that there is nothing inside us he did not already know of, by looking with such eyes and in such light as he has, he would be faced with more and more coming, as individuals do come, born every day and moving every day into responsible speech, and they too may say they are different. He would have to kill them each and all.

Our state—difference, as well as identity—is as much a fact of the world as the force of gravity. It is as ordinary as a fact can get. It is a "fact of life," as we say, in this world as it is. We know that denial of connection, connecting through to a point of identity, is a sickness and is ultimately our death. The lessons of the twentieth century have been hard lessons. But then, so is denial of difference a sickness and ultimately our death. What do we do with our *differ-*

ence, how do we live with it? We work, I think, each a source of the other, rather more than just a resource. We rouse ourselves and look and listen, and take in "all the mighty world" (in Wordsworth's fine line) "of eye and ear—both what they half create, and what perceive." The combination of difference and identity, and not just dogged combination but coherence and sanity and life, is achieved through assent one to another and one with another. "Achieved" is an active term—this is the work the world requires, but leaves it to us to genuinely want to do.

Chapter Eight

THE OPENING
AND THE LINE

And so we come to the task of understanding what is being said when total theories are presented by some of us to all of us, and we come to the very human desire for help—help even in understanding what is being said when what seems to be said is that there is never help, never real help, no real help anywhere in the universe.

FACTS LARGE AND SMALL: HUMAN LAW

There are other large facts with which to begin the task, beyond the necessity of assent, the presence of dissent. They are facts that also have to do with us and our presence, lying around us all the time, so familiar that they can be taken for granted and overlooked like the beating of one's heart. Or these may all be thought of as small facts, because they tend to be hidden. But each is a small fact on which much turns, like the diamond point beneath a spinning gyroscope.

One of these is of course law itself, the phenomenon of authority that links individuals and makes our joint life possible, as marvelous as the invisible hand of the economic system.

Think how often a ruler says or inscribes "I built" this church or that city or raised this great stone, or a modern chief executive says, "I turned this company around," or the papers and analysts say it for him. The ruler and the CEO laid no stone and pulled no rope. Hidden is agency, in which full human beings are responding to authority— and authority is responding to them, is indeed half-created by them. The theorist looking at an engraving of Pope Sixtus V erecting the obelisk at the center of St. Peter's Square, with ropes radiating out on all sides to eight hundred men, might wish to see forces running between the directing object (here the pope) and the mass of objects directed toward the stone. But those "forces" are the forces of authority. And while we who do not consider ourselves slaves (before, that is, we agree with those who may urge upon us that we are) do know from reports of slavery, or experience with the military, or reports or experience of twentieth-century totalitarianism, that much can be achieved through terror and training, we also suspect or know terror and training have close limits. The question whether and how much terror and training "explain" atrocity is at the heart of current arguments about the extent of responsibility for the Holocaust. Terror and training have close limits even in working with animals: there is a difference between the authoritative and the authoritarian there too, as the philosopher (and trainer) Vicki Hearne has so nicely brought to the attention of those of us who do not work with animals.[1]

Total theorists can imagine "commands" and "rules" backed by sanctions operating in the human world like rules and inexorable law in the world conceived in the descriptive and analytic disciplines. Physics and biology are full of the language of law, the "legitimate" and the "illegitimate." The ear alert to legal allusions is generally surprised at their frequency and centrality. There is what may be called a naiveté, about that which the theorist has thus brought over into his thinking on his own work; and when the theorist moves back into the human world, as a total theorist must, that naiveté becomes particularly striking.

Steven Weinberg's characterization of the "final laws of nature" we have already heard: "Knowing these laws, we would have in our possession the book of rules that governs stars and stones and everything else."[2] We have noted Jacques Monod's assumption of authority and law when he speaks of the "affliction . . . for all those among mankind who bear or will come to bear the responsibility for the way in which society and culture shall evolve," posed by

> societies . . . still trying to live by and to teach systems of values already blasted at the root by science itself. . . . [A]ll these systems rooted in animism exist at odds with objective knowledge, face away from truth, and are strangers and fundamentally *hostile* to science, which they are pleased to make use of but for which they do not otherwise care.[3]

Jean-Pierre Changeux, ending his *Conversations* by turning to ethics and the question whether "ethics may one day find itself elevated to the rank of a science," speaks of the "task of devising precise rules of conduct," "the various prescriptions that regulate behavior at a given moment of a history of a society," "the entire set of rules of interactions among the individual members of a social group," the "hierarchical and parallel sets of neurons [that] contribute to the cognitive functions that jointly construct a code of right action," "Darwinian variations of social representations . . . propagated from one brain to another, selected at the level of the community, and finally retained in the minds of lawmakers." (pp. 210–12, 216, 219, 231)

But in law commands are statements in human language, "rules" are statements in human language, made by persons, always open to challenge, always but one among many statements being read and heard by other persons choosing what to listen to and what not. Speakers speak over and over, fade in life, and are replaced by speakers who speak anew; listeners or readers read again and again, and are continuously replaced by new readers who read anew.

When anything approaching a "rule" is invoked, or a "command," the very substance of the statement depends upon whether the person speaking is read in good faith, or not in good faith, manipulatively, by a person, deciding later. "What is meant?" is the question constantly being asked by one who is deciding whether and how to act. Sixtus V,[4] "over" the eight hundred men at the ends of ropes prepared to spend the day raising the obelisk at St. Peter's, is said to have ordered the men to keep silence during the raising, on pain of death. He erected a gallows nearby and in sight to remind the men he meant it. But what was "it" that he meant? Halfway up, the ropes chafed with friction on the granite and were about to snap, when a workman finally cried out, "Water for the ropes," and the chafing was stopped and the obelisk was raised. The pope came over and congratulated the workman for speaking out. What did the pope mean when he ordered silence on pain of death?

But it is not merely an intellectual, a conceptual, a theoretical difficulty the large fact of law presents the total theorist when he turns to the human world. The theorist is *in* the human world. He must have the law, he does have the law; and since he must, and when he does, he turns a human face to those to whom he speaks of his cosmology, and his face is read, as is usual, along with his words.

TOTAL THEORY AND LAW

On this—on having to have law—let us recall that total theory is a theory not only of the theorist and of the language in which the theory is put, but (especially) a theory of the person to whom the theory is put.

"Human beings all have the same (or virtually the same) brain!" the neurobiologist Changeux insists in his *Conversations.* (p. 33) The mathematician Connes responds later, "The structure of the brain, as you've pointed out, isn't identical from one person to another." (p. 128) We may identify with another person; we may also, and at the same time, be king of ourselves and the last word on ourselves (though like the king in *Antigone,* it may be too lonely to have the last word if the word is only and nothing more than our own). We took this up when we touched on scientific method in chapter 7. There would be nothing mad and utterly dismissible about an individual saying to the theorist, "I am not like you, you at least as you seem to say you are, and I am not like your picture of me." Anyone, you or I, can say and believe that; at some level I imagine we do, whatever the picture drawn by another of yourself or himself may be: novels and poems continue to be written, and each may carry some revelation. And any of us could go on to say to the theorist with something close to a taunt, "You will never be able to satisfy yourself fully, because you cannot look inside me unless I allow you to."

Extend physical difference (the difference despite which we know we can identify and join) and imagine the total theorist a man and the resisting individual a woman. The theorist can seek to *persuade* her, that she is like him as he purports to see himself, and that she is like the picture he paints of her. But if he does seek to *persuade* her he acknowledges her and speaks beyond his theory.

Or he can force her to *do* one thing or another: he might take her arm and make it write what he wanted, like the backscratcher on his bureau, one of those with a little cupped hand at the end of it. But we can imagine that would be unlikely to satisfy him. He can perhaps force her to *say* one thing or another, including the string of words he has used in presenting his picture of her to himself and to her. This should not satisfy him any more than the taking of her arm to make it do something, though we know that something close to the forcing of *saying,* saying on pain of suffering of sanctions otherwise, has been part of education of the young.

Or the theorist can marginalize her, and himself try to forget her and prevent her from speaking to him or others if she interferes with his urging and satisfaction in his urging.

But if the theorist uses something other than the strength of his own arm or the power of his own voice to do any of these — *prevents* interference or *makes* her do or say or *excludes* her — he uses the law, and in his appeal to the law he acknowledges a being and a form of being beyond that which he wishes to press as containing everything.

We can go further and imagine the theorist, as we did before, moving not just to marginalize, exclude, prevent, or force another to do or say, but moving actually to look inside the one who taunts him saying she is different from him and different from his picture of her, and we can imagine her resisting the look inside. Entertain the thought that the line separating cosmology from atrocity might break but nonetheless law would remain with us, at least for a time, at least at the time the line is crossed toward "sacrifice" of a human being in the technological sense, the sense in which an experimental animal is sacrificed. If she resists and is prepared to resist to the death, the invader, the sacrificer, turns to authority, to law, and to all that authority implies and demands.

What the total theorist says and does and presupposes when he turns to law cannot escape us, nor escape the theorist when he is candid. If, not just in supposition but in fact, the line between song sparrow and child was broken and no longer seen, we cannot say how long the force of law would remain with us; moments, or months, or years. The question is one with which Lon Fuller gallantly struggled after the Second World War, thinking about the years of Nazi rule, in the center of high Western culture, and the appeals to law there.[5] It is a question raised in many ways by issues with which some are openly struggling today, issues newly presented by the availability of fetal tissue, the pressures of extended aging, the desire to engage in studies of medical treatments given without regard to the welfare of each individual being studied. We do not know what would happen to us, us including the theorist, and with the theorist the theory, if the line were no longer seen. The authority of law with us now does not just empower the theorist beyond the strength of his own arm, it protects the theorist against reprisal. We do not know, we cannot say. But Lewis Thomas's "saddest tale" should hover around us, song sparrows left to make an "unmelodious buzzing noise." The twentieth century is there now, rounded in the way we round centuries, for us to contemplate.

THE IMPORTANCE OF A THING

After the large fact of law, we might notice importance itself. The world is flat in total theory—the neurobiologist's world that we have had before us does not differ in this from the mathematician's. To the mathematician, something is more important than something else, deeper, more generative, more elegant, more comprehensive. But not to mathematics: the world of mathematical objects simply is. How ultimate can that world be, for the mathematician himself, or for us listening to reports of the mathematician's experience of elegance, beauty, comprehensiveness? It is the interest of mathematicians in mathematics that is so interesting, when its ultimacy is proposed.

In the competing vision we have seen, of a world of swirling flux from beginning to end or without beginning or end, in which all, including mathematics and the mathematician, becomes processes and processes of processes, system dissolving into system, things merely happen. The forces completely in charge bow ultimately to the processes that produce them, and the processes that produce them likewise bow to the processes that produced them unless they reach back, transform, absorb utterly as they proceed on. Things merely happen and nothing can be more important than anything else because it is merely something happening. There is no such thing as catastrophe. The raging fire that caught up with the smoke jumpers in Norman Maclean's *Young Men and Fire*[6] is grass burning. Grass burning is just something happening. Flesh burning is no different. The wind rises, the fuel changes, the temperature escalates, the spread accelerates, process builds on process, the organization of the fire replaces the organization of a tree, of a human body; and then the fire is gone.

Yet even among those who might bravely purport to see no difference between grass burning and flesh burning, no difference really whatever the tugs of sentimentality, there is such interest in the stabilities that occur in the course of process, interest in how stabilities can occur in the organization of units into which reality divides itself, or into which the processes of our perception have divided it.

Why is there such interest in these stabilities, in this world of flux and change? Why not step back a little further so that they can hardly be seen, choose a stretch of time so that they are offered to perception like a single flicker of a fire? Is this interest in little stabilities just chance? The systems, of which we consist, fitting like lock to key to stabilities as such? Anyone can entertain a hope that something like that could eventually be shown. But that seems so lame an explanation of the particular attention paid to the stabilities that seem to emerge from process—the interesting large fact of the interest itself that makes the flat landscape not flat despite avowal that it is. Something seems hidden. After all, what is reduced to system disappears as important at the same time it disappears as itself, as an individual human, or otherwise. Explaining by process and system is explaining "away."

Were we hedonists and only hedonists we might say that explaining away is a route to a particular pleasure, the pleasure of being finished and done with things that bother, finding a place for them in a procession that will take them away so that they are no longer with us. It is not flesh burning in a forest fire, not really. The young man is not more important or different really from the fire itself; and both will be gone. But there remains this (now small) fact of interest in stabilities, which does not go away. It is like a loose thread in one's shirt or sweater that one notices from time to time, snips off, but appears again: in a fabric of thought that is to cover everything everywhere and forever, a loose thread.

To return to the particular community of thought we have had as an example: there is within mathematics itself a noticing of this loose thread, a glancing at it. It will be remembered that in arguing with a mathematician over whether there is a mathematical reality transcending material systems and processes, the neurobiologist allied himself with what some call the "constructivists" among mathematicians, contrasting them with "realists" for whom there is a non-material reality. Constructivists purport to see mathematics as a cultural object and "mathematical objects" as entirely the product of mathematicians, the form nature takes for the moment at the intersection of processes "inner" and "outer," the outcome of an interaction between the physiology of the genetically developed and environmentally molded brain and "social" forces.

Some among mathematicians, spending their life engaged in mathematical inquiry, view this very vision as a threat to mathematics itself, a "cancer" threatening to destroy.[7] Why it should ever be thought a threat to the doing of mathematics, rather than merely a debate about what mathematics "is," is a pointer to this small fact, this large fact, always there, generally taken for granted. The fact is the fact of interest in doing mathematics, the *doing* of mathematics, with its ties to an interest in life, the continuing to live it. That intense pursuit, that long puzzling, that ignoring of other calls and sacrifice of other claims—this is what is noticed, glanced at. It has not died, it does not die. There is no letting processes, including processes working through oneself, go on as they will. There is an intervention, a molding, even of the processes operating through oneself.

Necessary illusion, it may be said. But the curious fact which we all know, which is almost the sign of our particular brotherhood and sisterhood, after (as it was put once) we ate from the tree of knowledge but were stopped before we could get to the tree of life, is that living is not necessary, acting rather than letting be is not necessary, struggling rather than letting go is not necessary.

And as for illusion, the question is what we conclude about the way things are; and here is this fact, that we do go forward, in mathematics, and elsewhere, which is evidence on which to base a conclusion and come to a belief about the way things are. If one cannot understand it as one explains things to oneself, one pushes on— one *does* push on—to another way of understanding. If there is no place in one's belief for this that one does not or cannot deny (cannot, and continue to live) then one digs more deeply into one's belief. Or into the belief of another whom one is listening to and does not turn away from.

THE PRESENCE OF GOOD FAITH

The fact of human law, the fact of importance itself, and then the presence of good faith in the world. Small or large as its presence may be thought to be, what we call good faith is a fact and an actively helping fact.

The experience in law with efforts to define good faith in a person and in a person's manner of approach, and to systematize it in rules, is as nice an example as any of the limit to definition and "rule," and of the living that is beyond them. Good faith is invoked in law in any number of contexts—firings of employees, termination or nonperformance of contracts, indemnification, partnership, fiduciary duty, claims of limited liability, compliance programs in organizations subject to the criminal law, securities disclosure, insurance, lawyer discipline for filing frivolous suits. The list is a very long one. If good faith is defined in some particular context or field in which it is invoked, then the discovery is made, and it is made again and again, that one without good faith, the manipulator, can by manipulation render the definitions of "good faith" transparent, ineffective where he is active. He can successfully "evade."

Language strains and pulls against this, of course. The drafter struggles. But in the end the best that can be said is that unless the definition of good faith is treated in good faith, the definition is not satisfied. Either good faith, "it," disappears when defined, or it requires good faith beyond its definition to survive, good faith un-defined. The definition does not capture good faith if it is compre-hensive. If it does work to achieve good faith, it is not comprehensive.

The scientist, like the legal drafter, seeks rules and components organized and governed by rules. The scientist manipulates his rules and his material, testing them both. But the scientist is not entirely a manipulator. Despite the object of the effort, we can point to the good faith the scientist shows toward other scientists, toward experi-mental method, toward the profession. If he does not, he is con-demned, actually and genuinely condemned, and not for breaking any rule that could be stated. Or there is laughter. If condemnation is put aside, he is simply not taken seriously. There are no rules for laughter, either; laughter dies as it is defined—or laughs at its defi-nition: laughing or hearing laughter is a sign one is at an opening.

Scientists, mathematicians, and historians all know and prac-tice good faith. They know what it is to enter into the spirit of a thing. They know and practice good faith even at the same time they may be pursuing a vision in which it has no place. Politicians, litigating lawyers, and advertisers may continue to be heard without regard to their good faith, operating in systems that make use of their words. But if scientists, mathematicians, or historians do not practice good faith, and make a persuasive claim that they do not in fact know what it is, they are soon not heard anymore.

CANDOR AND THE LINE

The candor of which we have spoken, something so relatively simple that might yet be so large a contribution and a help, is very close to good faith and is associated with it. The world, it seems, will not operate without systems and manipulation, without negotiation, strategy, bluff, feints, traps, triumph and defeat, without privacy and secrets indeed. It is not total candor that can realistically be asked. It is rather candor and help in understanding when "all" and "everything" appear in description, argument, and challenge. Think of Marx. Marx and Marx's texts give the twentieth century much of its distinctive flavor, both in what they generated and in what they evoked in response. It was an encounter with the totalitarian in thought as well as in action in Marxist Russia, based, it was said, upon science, that so shocked the chemist Michael Polanyi because it left no place for truth or the pursuit of science.[8] But it was Marx as well who exclaimed, "Let us assume *man* to be *man* and his relation to the world to be a human one. Then love can only be exchanged for love, trust for trust."[9] Only the "only" in that cry might a human being at the end of the twentieth century wish to take up with Marx the prophet if the century could be lived over again, at the same time "all" and "everything" were being taken up with Marx the scientist and historicist.

And bound up with good faith and candor, hardly distinguishable in practice from either, is recognition of the line, on this side of which we have put the child, and on the other the sparrow. Human beings at the end of the experience of the twentieth century might want to emphasize this most, if the century could be lived over again.

Not "all" is on this side of the line. We do not know even whether the world can operate without putting some human beings across the line into cages or killing human beings by war or neglect. But not "all" is on the other side of the line. At least some things are treated in good faith and approached in good faith, some human beings at some times, if not all at all times, even some texts, or ventures like science, or what we call institutions. They are not to be used, or not to be only used, not to be merely manipulated, and not to be destroyed—not without suffering in doing so, which is itself recognition of a limit.

What of the example of total theorists and the pictures they paint of themselves? Beyond his evident respect for science, Jean-Pierre Changeux can say of individuals in the world with him that drug addiction is "tragic" and war "absurd madness."[10] It is when he turned to his cosmology that we heard him say any belief of his "may be defined as a specific state of nerve cell activity . . . that can propagate from one brain to another, and spread 'infection' much as viral attacks do, suggesting comparison with epidemics." (*Conversations,* p. 227) He moves from animal to child: "Suturing the eyelid over one eye of young monkeys . . . sharply modifies the functional specificity of the neurons of the visual cortex—a result that probably applies to other regions of the brain, the frontal cortex in particular. . . . Beliefs and moral rules are fixed simultaneously, and perhaps in analogous ways, with the acquisition of a native language. The child's brain becomes impregnated with moral rules, as it were, along with a language. . . . The neurocognitive basis for the establishment of beliefs remains unknown for the most part, of course. It will furnish the basis for a good deal of fascinating research in the years to come." (p. 221) Again, we heard John Searle tell us that as a total theorist he lives in "a world that consists entirely of physical particles in fields of force." "Systems," he said, "are collections of particles where the spatio-temporal boundaries of the system are set by causal relations," and after referring to small raindrop and large glacier as each a system, he too brings in the human child and puts the child beside the animal and the inanimate, like raindrop beside glacier: "Babies, elephants, and mountain ranges are also examples of systems."[11]

Fascinating, the question of language and belief. How *does* the child come into language, this very language that is being used to speak to us of suturing eyelids and systems and visions of the world, to speak to us of language itself? The song sparrow sings. The young song sparrow learns to sing, and comes to sing his own song. Whence comes any real reluctance in total theorists to treat the child like the young song sparrow, deafening him, keeping him in silence, isolating him, sacrificing him, and cutting his brain into slices?

But taking all in all, the reluctance is real, not strategic, not a hesitation total theorists would free themselves of if they could— taking all in all, listening to all that is said by those who urge such visions of the world, watching them live, summoning them in mind to stand in front of the monitors at the Holocaust Memorial Museum, and looking into their eyes.

Chapter Nine

THE CLAIM OF THE CHILD

THE OPENING AND THE LINE

What there is through the opening in system and process my words cannot fill, and I cannot fill alone.

So many paintings of landscape are of openings, with light or a horizon beyond. And so much of the twentieth century's abstract art. The opening beyond may be the secret of the allée, the garden vista small or large, the garden path, even the angled row of trees on a hillside or the columns we still put in rows, wordlessly bringing to mind our experience and place in the world.

Could miracle step through the opening? Why yes, I suppose it could—it would be called miracle, because it, whatever it was, stepped through the opening to join us in reality.

But "miracle" is so freighted a term that using it may put too high a price on candor. For some, mathematics goes beyond or is beyond, steps through, escapes process if not system, and joins direct experience, as real as anything is real. The uncanny which is the shadow of miracle is as close as mathematicians generally want to come—or as far as they want to go—in explicitly describing mathematics' place in experience. For some, Mary steps through—but "stepping through" is a useful way of talking, of becoming explicit, only if it is remembered that there is something of a stepping through at once in both directions: stepping through from the beyond to us, what comes back to us as we look at the opening in a painting; stepping through, figure, voice, fire, from system and process to us beyond, for we are in systems, and systems are in us.

For some it is music, that is not mathematical—or eternally repeated. And for all, I think, there is much mundane through that opening there always is in systems' and processes' tightly woven and tightly wrapping fabric—much never thought miraculous or even strange because so familiar. There is death of course, the shortness of life. So little time, only a taste, a glimpse of the world. "Short" we noticed before is without place in a world of system where there is only difference. It is defined in fact by disappointment and dissatisfaction—were we not dissatisfied with the time we have, life would be long enough—which disappointment and dissatisfaction again have no place in a form of thought that coolly sees all as system. Speak of death, stand up and uncover the head in respect for death, and you have stepped through the opening, something has come to you through the opening.

The individual too, whose death it is. Language itself. The land, of which Wendell Berry is singing as I write. Such experience can be ordinary and open to large numbers of us, "common" if not universal. It can show variety that only travel and long talk reveals. It is whatever there is of meaning or value in the processes that fascinate and carry us along. Or, we might equally say, it is whatever there is of spirit in the processes and systems of the world, "spirit" a word not too parochial to use because it is used by those who would deny it.

We live in a world of reports back from our fellows. This alone may make impossible, forever, any vision that could identically fill the mind and all the mind of every one of us who comes and goes. Some of us struggle long to express and all of us know what the struggle is to express what we sense on our own; and the forms of expression, the means of expression, the metaphors, are always changing. The new always astonishes, in ordinary life no less than in the mathematical world Alain Connes found inexhaustible. For Ortega y Gasset, "living means dealing with the world, turning to it, acting in

it, being occupied with it." Then, sounding rather like a "string theorist" in physics searching during his working day for a final theory,
whose particular assumptions Ortega would most certainly challenge,
he continues, "That is why man is practically unable, for psychological reasons, to do without all-round knowledge of the world, without
an integral idea of the universe."[1] But as Blake advises in his "Now I
a fourfold vision see,"[2] I suspect all do live and (given the large fact
that all depend upon reports and respond to them) must live with
multiple visions, akin to the at least twofold vision of the good doctor,
of whom the Lewis Thomas with whom we began may be taken as
an example, bound to the individual, devoted to life, and exquisitely
sensitive to the working of systems and processes.

I suspect too that the entertaining of any absolute assumption
of connection between visions (or translation of one into another)
may be no more than the temporary elimination of one of them. It
may be of great importance to manipulate verbally units of reference in the material world, whether units of chemistry or money. It
may be equally important in the human world not to speak in a language of boxes.

But while the path to and from the opening, and what in its
whatness comes or goes down that path, none of us can perhaps
ever fully know now or in the future, the very fact that we can recognize gifts, value them rather than ignoring them as we ignore a
shutter banging in the wind, suggests that visions of the world are not
so fractured. The very fact that we listen to, try to understand, do
understand reports through language of what we cannot experience
directly or experience so well, suggests this. To be sure, given the
immediacy of the processes of the world, and given the individual
within us and before us and the person who can never be wholly
absorbed into the individual, a simple double-dwelling (within processes and beyond them) may not be a possibility, nor what might
seem the comparative restfulness of it. But still the world, in the
end and candidly faced, need not be a wilderness, a dark forest forever. At the least the multiplicity within us need not be a multiplicity
among us, the dreaded arbitrary and unreachable "subjectivity," from
which the only refuge is an "objectivity" in which the person has no
place. The fact is that we do speak to one another, and continue to

speak, and to listen. We do not always turn away from listening and do not always fall into silence and retreat from speaking as not worthwhile—rather, we seek to find some other way, including gesture and action that may speak in their own fashion, wordlessly. And as if that were the natural thing to do, there is not much pause or self-searching before we turn to other ways. We do not, that is, think of ourselves as saying "czpts" or "oqpt" to others, or of others as making such marks or sounds and offering them to us. In the same way those who would quip that the limbic system secretes love and the brain secretes thought as the liver secretes bile do not, when challenged on "love," respond that the challenger is saying "xqst." Both continue to argue about "love," and the moment one would say finally to the other that meaningless sounds are coming out of his mouth produced by environmental, cultural, and genetic systems, discussion would stop. But discussion does not stop.

Even those who might want discussion to stop find, as we have seen, that they are only individuals and must come back and appeal, for assent and support, for protection from others and effectuation through others. More, they must appeal not just one to one, but to human law—at some point they must in order simply to continue life and work. And, appealing, they do abandon a wholly manipulative stance, and do move authentically into the stance in which there can be a revelation in a single word.

INTIMATION

Back and forth goes the talk, the gesture, and the action, and so long as it does (which it does) individuals are not travelers coming back from distant lands bearing the wholly unrecognizable. Though they may not be dealing in common coin, their minds and worlds filled utterly by identical visions and understandings, still they are not offering one another—*we* are not offering one another—meaningless sounds and gestures, proffering stones rather than bread to each other's indicated hunger. We work with intimation from the beginning. Without it we plunge on, inattentive, uncaring. If we are attentive and take care, intimation however faint is there within us. We may not want to acknowledge it, may want to escape the thought it is there and the implications of the thought. But if we are candid with ourselves, shake ourselves and ask ourselves whether what we say and what we attend to really is insane, foolish, or false—if we read this evidence of ourselves that can be laid before us as much as evidence of another is laid before us—intimation is there with us. We work with intimation from what others say and do. We work from intimation to what we say and do.

We have actual knowledge of the least that can be said, the quietest thing, which our language might cast in the negative: we know what cannot be, even if we do not think we can say what is. We know that a vision or claim rising in us or received from another is inadequate or wrong, without having in hand a substitute for it that would be adequate and right. Intimation we experience in what our language might cast in the positive, as hint. Direct experience it seems, but experience of a suggestion, unshakable but still only suggestion, like evidence that a visitor has been with us whom we did not see. Much metaphor in writing, phrase or fragment in music, gesture in dance or in love goes no further than this. It has the same quality whether it is drawn from one's own experience and conveyed—for confirmation, or as help or as offering and gift—or is conveyed to one from another's experience. Hint may come, and hint may be conveyed, in the form of a question as in Jane Kenyon's lines now sung as part of a song cycle by William Bolcom:[3]

> These lines are written
> by an animal, an angel,
> a stranger sitting in my chair;
> by someone who already knows
> how to live without trouble
> among books, and pots and pans . . .
>
> Who is it who asks me to find
> language for the sound
> a sheep's hoof makes when it strikes
> a stone? And who speaks
> the words which are my food?

The capacity to ask a question is telling. An explanation of the question that does not offer an answer is never sufficient to make vanish the question of whether the explanation itself is enough.

Or the touch may be stronger than what we call intimation, leaving more than a question. There may be perception that leads to more than suggestion, to assertion or a report back that is of a vision, of sight and insight, of experience as direct as the experience of a stone on the foot or the digital readout of a spectrometer. This, which is matter of degree, may change with time of life. What can now be only suggested can later be confidently asserted; and what is seen young can be experienced when old only as suggestion, and with the crutch of memory—though still inescapable.

Such confident knowledge and the capacity for assertion is the happier state for the individual, to be hoped for before death. It is not the usual state. The usual, from reports by others of themselves, and observation of others, and reports of others of their observation of others, and reports they have from others (all put together in anyone's sense of the "usual" state of being human), is a grounded faith. Whatever the degree of conscious reflection and deliberate categorization of experience there may be—and it varies enormously—the usual would seem reflected in the use and appearance of "faith" in everyday language, from "good faith" to being "faithful" to another person, or animal, or to a joint undertaking, like experimental science.

INDIVIDUALITY AND KNOWLEDGE

We can imagine that the happy and hoped-for state of confident assertion would divide us from one another. It might tempt the use of force to extract confirming declarations, or to suppress or destroy sources of denial or doubt, or to monopolize the molding of minds in schools or through public utterance. But we cannot be absolutely certain it is confident knowledge that has fueled the use of force to produce speech or to suppress speech. Force can produce only the sounds of words in the air or prevent the sounds of words. The more truly confident the sight, the less need there is for declared confirmation; the less confident, the less there is within to sustain action against resistance or retaliation, and the more need there is for help and authentic confirmation, which can never be secured by forcing the sounds of some words out to reverberate in the air, or by eliminating human talk. Attributing the evils of history, and the cruelties of human beings one to another which so constantly astonish, to the human hunger for meaning rather than other kinds of hunger involves more often than not (like the evil and the cruelty itself) a slipping away or a deliberate turning away from meaning. The turn when meaning is actually in sight is toward its expression, so that its traces will be left upon the life of the seeing individual that continues on, to be re-evoked in its semblance, or remembered; and as a gift to be brought to others, in some exchange as it were for their own gifts. Though the expression, the means—the music, the language, the gesture, the action—may lead to another's direct sight of the same, any understanding that the gift had led to sight, that others actually saw by reason of such expression, would be based upon a report from those others, expression back in their turn. And the usual, again the usual, is that it is not the sight or insight itself that is conveyed, like a package across a divide, but an intimation of it; and the report back from others who received the gift is of intimation. One is oneself inevitably an intermediary between what one has seen, that "what," and others around one in this world. Each, in a way, is a priest to the other. This is not a texture of things where division grows.

Moreover if talk continues it melts the edges of any exclusivity of insight. To understand at all another's expression of what he says he knows and is there to be known, one may already have, have to have, an inkling of it oneself. To value mathematics and support mathematicians, rather than simply ignoring them as huddles of gibbering souls, one has a sense of mathematics. If it is not a direct taste of mathematical insight, it is a taste of what mathematical insight is like.

And this is not to say that one *must* have a sense of the thing. One does have. Valuing it and support of it is evidence of an inkling of what it is. This is true even of anything we tolerate and intervene to protect rather than overriding or leaving to lose its struggle. Toleration in the smallest way, that one protects it from oneself and one's indifferent crushing as one crushes blades of grass when one walks, is evidence. By virtue of the very fact we so single it out from the blades of grass beneath our feet and all that we pass by indifferently, we are partway to understanding, however small the part.

The fact that others may see more (if this were a matter for quantification) or see better (if this were a matter of competition) no more raises threat of the division and fracturing of humanity than the fact that some can love better, which we can understand because we know at least something of what love is, and which we can welcome. More filaments of the vicarious connect us than we can unravel or count. The dancer and the athlete leap and turn a graceful torso for the awkward and the injured, and it might not be enough for the dancer and the athlete to leap just for themselves. The gifted mathematician and musician may bless the presence of the most ordinary person who is full of life, and envy that fullness of life, as itself a gift.

And all the assurance in the world, all the coalescence of confirmations that might begin to pull an individual away from this participation in the variety of individual experience, cannot avoid the necessity of assent that we have touched upon before. Not one of the collective "positions" taken on what is beyond, on the largest things on which one takes a position, speaks with one voice. "Christianity," "Islam," "Judaism," "Hinduism," "Buddhism" each offer a variety of view, in the same way "science" or "mathematics" does on the largest things on which one takes a position. There is that same absence of unanimity that makes "antiscience" so difficult a position to maintain—because one must oneself construct the "science" to be against—even as the same absence makes an appeal to "science" so difficult for the total theorist.

We may ask whether there is a soul of Islam, Christianity, Buddhism, or any other credal effort to gather in what enters through the opening in the systems and processes of the world. But that would be for any of us to say—or as many of us who can talk together in the short time we have to talk. But we could not say, unless those reaching for the word "Islam" or "Christianity," in their own efforts to express, are listened to, actually listened to, and not treated as engines driven by "motivations" closed to us except as forces that can be externally defined and categorized for insertion into a vision of emerging and disintegrating systems.

We have asked whether there is a soul of "science," or of "mathematics." Is mathematics which is beyond process different from music? Is music, including the music that mathematicians are so often drawn to love and play, different from the music of the spheres? Look around and pick up this claim here, that claim there. Are mathematics, music, language, Mary, Torah, Buddha offered as a thing itself that is beyond? I myself do not think so, but any of us can listen to what is being said. If they are offered as means to, outposts of—what? Let us use the word "spirit" again until talk can go beyond it: are they each an outpost, hint in themselves, of a spirit or the spirit? Are they each a waypath to a spirit or the spirit? Is love a means, or the thing itself? Outpost, if outpost it is, of a spirit or of the spirit? Again we listen, and go on listening, in this fascinating world where we all discover, as time runs out, that we have been given surprisingly little time.

ALIKENESS AND THE LINE

We ask, we listen, we go on listening. What can we ourselves say, from within the extraordinariness of our individuality, about being human?

What I think we can all say is that the variety of which we hear report does not fracture us within or separate us. Not only because it does not *seem* to us, as we continue to talk and listen without throwing up our hands at our own foolishness in doing so, that we are in a situation where some are seeing what others cannot see anything of at all; but because where hint and intimation are what is experienced and conveyed, there is indicated but left unstated what intimation is intimation of. And variety, whatever we say our experience of it is, does not fracture us, as humanity, or separate us as total theory does, or would if it were believed—separating purported believer in it from those who see it as a crudeness of thought, and separating us all as we would be separated if we were pulled back across the line where we would be things, not persons, units fungible and silent, not individuals speaking and being listened to. Whatever our experience of variety, we have the common experience of looking into the eyes of others as eyes of fellows and companions, and of trusting that others are looking at us in the same way. When we do look and see, a sense of life springs within us—this is when the words "we live" can be uttered fully meaning them. At the point where a person is seen, actually seen, there can be a falling back almost as from a surprise, the mind filled, and such encounters can be experienced with individuals slow-witted, maddened, twisted. Great care, great care, counsels common experience, before any final declaration that someone is just deficient.

We each and all have this direct experience at the least, of seeing a person and being seen as a person. It is the experience that keeps us together. We also know what it is to see another not as a person, and how that affects our action. How we see others—and ourselves—makes "all the difference in the world," the difference that there is, in the world, between what is on one side of the line, and what is on the other. We can blink, and the person before us is on the other side of the line. We can blink again, and he is with us here again.

Perhaps children with their parents or in schoolyard crowds practice this, seeing others around them as animal, different and unreadable, with snouts for noses and paws for hands—seeing in clapping, for instance, not applause but the banging of paws together—then in a trice blinking them back to the human. As adults we experiment with crossing the line in perception and in action during the daily administration of the criminal law. At sentence to prison a person goes through a door and on the other side becomes a thing. His individuality is deliberately taken from him. His name is replaced with a number, the treatment of his hair he has chosen is shorn away, his body is put into a uniform and his clothes are taken. He is made fungible. The repetition of routine is that of a machine part, a system in operation. Communication with him is not possible, blocked by a material wall. He is introduced to a meaningless silence, where the sounds that do ripple through the air are only to push him to physical motion or to restrain, and he is to respond to them as a stick responds to the ripples of a wave. No one cares about him. No one is interested in hearing the sounds he makes.

Thus, mirroring exactly the features of modern total theory as if we all along have known what it was, is a stretch of his life taken from him, when he cannot say "I live." If there is the death penalty, he is eventually killed, and his face will be covered before he is killed so that no one can look into his eyes.

Modern criminal punishment *is* being put on the other side of the line. Such justification as is offered for it makes it a consequence of the convict's himself ignoring value and himself putting human beings on the other side of the line. We are familiar as well with the restoration, a recrossing of the line that, if it is fully a stepping back, involves something more than release from prison and the "former" convict growing his hair, assuming his name, putting on his clothes, and becoming an individual again. To be spoken to as before, and listened to as before, there enters what we call remorse on the one side, and forgiveness on the other.

Pushing away, across the line between system and person, closing the opening to person and to us where we live, and taking back— "saving" is perhaps the word for it still, which says also how ancient the experience and the problem are. Moving in thought and action from "we" to "you" to "it," and then from "it" to "you" to "we" (pronouns contain so much). Pushing away, embracing. While, again, I am but one individual and cannot think in principle or outline all the variety there can be once the limit of system and process is reached and acknowledged, this work at the line, thought affecting action, action revealing thought, does seem very close to a common human experience that can be encountered by anyone however situated.

What total theory proposes, if it were read as if believed, is ourselves following what we push across the line, and never coming back. This is the import of theory that encompasses the theorists themselves as well as those to whom they speak it and the language in which they speak it. Speculation about the consequences is more a matter of exploring inchoate folk memories of the century just closed than offering orderly and articulate propositions for testing. History and social commentary fall silent before the enormities and the revelation of their real possibility, categories failing, words inadequate. The inner limit on the span of a regime of true evil, the implosion of the truly evil mind, may be a matter of faith and never demonstrable, may be treated really only in novel and story because none of our available disciplines reach it any more than they reach evil itself. But it seems that those responsible for twentieth-century totalitarian thought and action, treating others as the mere products of systems and as material to be manipulated or eliminated, did begin to think of and treat themselves in the same way, as not responsible because there is no responsibility but only system and process. Then collapse and destruction follow, either through individual madness or ultimate isolation with each the enemy of the other, or (a lawyer might observe) through the collapse of authority, and the joint effort that depends upon authority, when appeal to the person can no longer be made.

This is one consequence of treating "all" as things not to be listened to, nor the hand stayed against them. Alternatively, *all* are not in fact thought about and treated in this way, because those responsible for such thought and action do not think about and treat themselves in this way. Then there can be an appeal to candor. In the reverse of the infection that spreads back to themselves from the way totalitarians treat others, the way in which totalitarians treat themselves, responsible, individual, facing death and seeking meaning, can spread out to others.

It is the postulate and basic belief we are alike—or not alone—that plucks so at the fabric of total theory. We have tried here to approach human likeness, and the human claim, through the necessity of assent and through the revelations of language and of action and of staying the hand, without putting aside the newness of individual experience and report. Criminal condemnation, this common experience of what the line means in action, is understood as maintaining this perception of likeness, insofar as it is understandable at all other than as wrenching tragedy. Those who push others across the line in punishment do so in an avowedly responsible way, albeit speaking for the law—in the West, it is judge and jury, prosecutor with public obligations, court of appeal, executive declining clemency. It is punishment, this treatment of human beings, and not mere "treatment," because the convicted too are responsible. The nature of the punishment, the state of existence into which the convicted enter, is a designed contrast between responsibility and the absence of responsibility. At least before the point where a declared criminality has shaded into mind-numbing evil, there remains an identification with the condemned, and acknowledgment that crime is possible for the normal and that the condemning might someday be the condemned; and it is this that places some limit on punishment, its length, its nature, stretched though that limit is and surprisingly horrible what is done within it. Criminality, after all, that in the United States can alone constitutionally justify such punishment, turns not on the occurrence of some physical event in the world, nor upon "breaking" a "rule," but on the presence of mind, what in legal terms is called the "mind of the accused" or *mens rea*.

There is, to be sure, an interweaving of the criminal with worlds in which the human fades away. For medical experimentation on human subjects in the United States, thought turns to the prison.[4] Before entering the Gulag in Russia, or before Chinese entered the laboratories to become "logs" for medical experimentation in Japanese-occupied Manchuria, there generally were convictions, the forms of criminal law observed before pushing human beings across the line to where consent becomes irrelevant and voice is silenced. And there is, of course, capital punishment from which there is no return. But despite this interweaving, there is a sense that things can go too far and a restlessness when they do; and it is a general sense, flowing from our ordinary ability to blink others and perhaps ourselves back and forth across the line.

MADNESS AND THE LINE

What is not so common, but still accessible as experience of the line, is the declaration and treatment of insanity in others. Connected with it is the temporary or not so temporary participation in what is called atrocity (in revulsion against it, after the fact), which is also called madness, but madness not on the part of those no longer listened to, rather madness on the part of those who no longer listen.

Law is necessarily involved in the encounter with insanity, and therefore are all those involved who participate in decisions that have force derived from the authority of law. Insanity is a matter for medicine, and for novelists and painters, but also for jurors, judges, and lawyers because a claim of it moves so often to one individual seizing hold of another identified as human by himself or herself, or by others, seizing not his money or his things but his body. Insanity—for those who must face it and make decisions with respect to it—is a disappearance of the person from sight, a movement further and further away, to the point where the postulate or underlying belief of alikeness is almost severed and one's effort to understand, to listen, to hear another, or to take into account that other's reading of one-self (in understanding oneself), comes to an end.

Mystery though insanity remains (in law or elsewhere), and beyond "definition" quite as much as good faith is beyond definition, there has been less inclination to see the insane as a being "possessed," a "holy fool," and more to see the insane as diseased, insanity as a "syndrome," the product of systems and processes that are, ultimately, only to be explained and, as systems only, to be manipulated if possible. The very desire to manipulate, rather than ignore or destroy if bothersome, bespeaks a residual identification with this that was once perceived as a person. Insanity, "abnormal" by contrast to the "normality" of the criminal, most people sense is not an absolutely impossible state for themselves: there is *recognition* of it. But while the desire to manipulate, to care and cure, hangs on a thread of identification—and what may still remain of an ancient sense of possession and mystery—the willingness to manipulate grows as the sense grows stronger that sound, cry, look, movement, gesture, action are the products of processes and only the product of processes within the body that has been seized.

There is no anger at the processes or at the insanity or at the insane. There is no condemnation of them. There could not be, any more than there really could be anger at a firestorm in a valley, at the firestorm itself. If anger or condemnation erupt, they are checked, as foolish, inappropriate, out of place, impossible.

But the discovery has been, by those involved in authorizing the movement of some individuals against others on grounds of insanity, that once the declared insane have been put on the other side of the line, they have been treated in the same way as convicts, if not somewhat worse: to correction by what otherwise would be called assault, to injection with drugs, to deprivation of light, warmth, hygiene. None of this was punishment, any more than caging an animal or injecting it or castrating it or hitting it is really punishment of the animal, not punishment however similar it was to the treatment of the criminal after he passed through the door of the courtroom and his clothes were replaced with a uniform. But there was no forgiveness either. Forgiveness was as irrelevant as condemnation or anger. And there was no end to it. No bounded part of a life could be taken because there was, in the sense in which we say "we live" or "she is full of life," no life here to take a part from, only the "life" of the processes called disease.

As a result of this discovery, from the mid-twentieth century on[5] those participating in responsibility for justifying by the authority of human law the treatment of the declared insane have pulled back from discussing insanity as disease in the same way as flu is discussed as disease. There is today a sense of dilemma. In an exemplary way it is empirically based, upon our experience of our own behavior in the twentieth century, our experience of the line and the effect of thought on action.

Of the other experience of putting the human on the other side of the line that might be deemed a special legacy of the twentieth century, there is much debate over its breadth and depth. How deep into belief was thinking a large part of the population of Europe "vermin" suitable for working to death or extermination?[6] How common was the thought, how common action upon it? What was the experience, of training, of thinking after training, and of acting upon thinking, that makes American veterans of the Vietnam War so apparently different from veterans of other wars? For they are more troubled. The presence of dissent and a challenge to the righteousness of the war, a mere difference of view from what had to be their own view as they fought, seems inadequate as a source of their own special troubledness. Then there is the experience of the other twentieth-century wars, participated in by as many as have marched in the ranks of armies. Active experience of war eventually involves placing populations, and individuals suddenly close-confronted from among them, at least partially across the line "as if" they were ants, automatons, figures of wood, for purposes of death and gross forms of manipulation, if not (today) torture or slavery. Other human beings are separated and made different from those in the ranks acting thus "as if," often by no more than a declaration, called a "Declaration of War," that can appear in the space of a blink, and can be blinked back again so that the opposing ranks suddenly break and rush forward to embrace and rejoice. But even this partial or limited pushing across the line, the half-believed "as if," is generally acknowledged in reflective peace to be a "temporary madness."

Such a state of perception of other human beings is aided and perhaps engendered by the perceiver's himself being made a reflection of that which is on the other side of the line, only system, only process, oneself a nameless and fungible unit, taking the form of a unit by being encased in what we call a "uniform," and responding without personal responsibility to the mere force of sounds that stimulate or restrain physical movement. Obey, not as to human law but as "obedience" is to a "law" of nature; do not speak back; act as part of a system; remove awe, fear, and respect for death, for death has no place in the operation of systems—there is only a recombination and replacement of units.

This is the way the sane view the insane, save that now one is viewing oneself in this way. The way one has been asked or trained to view others, the enemy, has crept back across the bridge of alikeness and become the way one views oneself. And it is the residual sense this is not all one is that makes the "madness" of war only temporary, with candor about oneself spreading across the bridge of alikeness again into one's sense of others. "Total war" is a vision of the human world that has absorbed into it a vision of the cosmos in which there is no place for the human; but then this is peculiarly the lesson of the century, this linkage between various experiments with the total.

As for individual atrocity, not systematized or depending on system, there is not common experience. Nor would it seem in any way peculiar to the twentieth century. It merges back into individual crime, though the very term "atrocity" pushes against the threads of identification with the perpetrator that limit punishment. How many babies have been tossed in the air and caught on bayonet, sword, or spear? How many babies' heads have been smashed against walls with their mothers watching? Enough to emphasize for those who do not think themselves personally capable of doing this a connection between action and perception of a certain kind. Anyone putting himself imaginatively in the position of the man tossing the baby up thinks first that the man cannot be seeing this child as like his own child. For him, this that he is spearing and smashing is spawn, roe. Those rounding up children, as such, in France for shipment off for medical experimentation spoke to themselves and others in these terms.[7] Not a child, but a bit of roe from a species. Not a child, but a genetic efflorescence, like an efflorescence of algae. Not a child, but in the eyes of the tosser, at the moment of the tossing, a property of a reproducing system. If the vision were blinked away while the baby was in the air, the arms that tossed the baby up would catch and cradle it as it came down.

And when the man returns to his own baby, and looks? Then candor may be too much to bear. The vision haunts. It too has a sword. In milder form, its sword still sheathed, it haunted even the gentle and generous Lewis Thomas.

Chapter Ten

THE CLAIM OF
THE SPARROW

THE CONTINUITY OF THE HUMAN

Science and antiscience. There need be no such division, and as a matter of fact there is not when we read one another closely, read ourselves closely, and attend to others' readings of us.

Working scientists need have no fear of others, only of others' misunderstanding. Others need have no fear of working scientists, because working scientists are themselves others. We are many, we are each here only a short time (or so it seems of others, and of ourselves if we are like others), and being utterly alone is not what we generally see as an object of life. Most work for the sake of others in the short encounter of each with this universe in which we are situated. In their very speaking of their experience of it they are speaking for the sake of others. This is as true for those working and speaking as scientists as for those who do not spend their lives in what they or others would call science.

Each in fact brings gifts, however beguiling it may be to talk of human affairs as if there were really no giving and really only taking. The ultimate, after taking all, in a world in which there is only taking, is utter, utter loneliness. This small fact feeds much of our actual view of each other, and of the nature of the universe in which we are situated. All bring gifts, and despite the fearful lessons of the twentieth century about our capacities and the consequences of our yearnings, or perhaps because of these lessons, we can hope for a time in which there are no martyrs, a time which will be neither the time of Nero nor the time of Galileo. Should such times of martyrdom come, we can hope both scientists and nonscientists would join to pull us all through them.

The joining would be in common allegiance to the empirical and to openness. During the experience of the twentieth century the spirit of scientific work has been the refuge and resting place for the sense and hope of progress. However the possibility of true progress may be viewed in the twenty-first century, there can at least be a joining in a hope of a more mutually sensitive empiricism and a more mutually sensitive openness, seeing what is there before us and within us, and listening to our reports of what we see that we offer to one another.

The rational can in no way be identified with the total. Nor can it be identified by contrast with the emotional. The good scientist has a passion for truth. We see that passion so clearly in the second Monod, the Monod of the end of *Chance and Necessity* speaking of "transcending the self to the point even of justifying self-sacrifice if need be." (p. 178) It is merely one instance of the connection between emotion and its object, joy *in,* love or hatred *of,* which draws emotion in its actuality away from the definition of it used in clinical and pathological study. Emotion blends with value; value with the presence of a person; person with action in the world—or restraint of action, with which we have been especially concerned here.

If an empirical cast of mind is what most of us most mean by rational—being open to evidence, being willing to shake irrelevance, being always willing to return to the reality of experience— then the candor to which we can look with hope is no embrace of the irrational. It is embracing the rational. If the joint use of mathematical insight and scientific method were the limit of the rational and "rationality" the word were to be pocketed by one method and form of thought, rationality would have a limit, a front edge, where reality cannot be encapsulated into units that can be put into systems, where the empirical is alive and bursts the confines of category and escapes all efforts to grapple it into a "feature" or "property." No matter how complex the systems that may be imagined and no matter how much their behavior may be seen as unpredictable and uncontrollable, systems and "system" itself cannot reach all that there is and that we experience even in our short lives, much less all of what others tell us of their experience.

Rationality need not be so limited, and is not so limited. Human language, that good scientists and good mathematicians speak as well as nonscientists and nonmathematicians, is full of this life which some part of each of us may wish to capture and hold but which in time we know and may candidly say we cannot capture. "Spirit" is the word used most generally for this that cannot be fully possessed and cannot be fully grasped but is no less real for it. In its contribution to the sense of being alive, to "I live!" coming from each of us, it is all the more real for being beyond the limits we create and feel and see. The spirit of a thing, the spirit of an action, the spirit of what we are talking about, and ultimately, the spirit of a person. To use the word "spirit" positively, and confidently: this is where candor leads, to spirit, at least to this, and from this we can proceed in our further exploration of the systems of the world in which we find ourselves, the scientist in all no longer shadowed by the antiscientist in any.

THE MOVEMENT OF THE LINE

Not even a fundamental desire to integrate man and nature, the human and the nonhuman, need divide us.

Lewis Thomas, with whom we began, expresses that driving desire from beginning to end in his appeals to nonscientists from the world of scientific work. We have seen example after example, Changeux, Monod, Jacob, Weinberg, state it in one form or another. To speak like John Searle of human beings as being "continuous" with nature may be only another way of presenting a total theory of system and process. But Searle would stay his hand from vivisecting a human being or pulling out a dog's nails with pliers and then burning it alive, and not merely, we may think, out of prudent deference to the superstitions of others. In staying his hand he would reveal much.

We have spoken throughout of the "line" between the song sparrow and the child, how the same questions can be asked about the child's development of auditory and musical capacities to the point where he has his own song, as can be asked about the song sparrow's development toward song; and how for the child, investigation waits for experimental evidence to present itself: a deaf child, a child that has been locked away, a child that dies for whom an autopsy can be authorized. But for the song sparrow, as even Lewis Thomas recounts, young are taken from their parents, deafened, reared in silence, sacrificed so that their brains can be sliced and examined. The line between the two is a line of action and restraint, that runs through value, significance, spirit, suffering, and death. That line can move.

It can be progressively erased, vanish in perception so that there is a continuity between the human and the nonhuman. But then either you deafen the child, or you do not deafen the sparrow. Why is the groan of an animal not a groan of suffering? Why is what is done by human hand to the animal to produce the groan not torture? Because of the line. Remove the line and it may become torture. Torturers of human beings, after all, need not be sadists. They are seeking something. They may be using suffering to achieve it, but doctors may use suffering too in their work. It is indifference to suffering as suffering, recognizable as suffering, that marks torture, that and indifference to the individual being used.

Recall the responses we noted at the end of chapter 5 to Steven Weinberg's summation, "The more the universe seems comprehensible, the more it also seems pointless." "Why should it have a point?" the astronomer Margaret Geller commented. "What point? It's just a physical system, what point is there? I've always been puzzled by that statement."[1] So might there be puzzlement about breaking open a rock, putting dirt in a furnace, poisoning slime, cutting a log, if it were asked whether this was torture. There is not just a mere convention of swearing in using "dirt," "slime," or "dumb as a log" as pejoratives and the strongest terms of abuse. It is not an entirely arbitrary choice of words that makes "dirt," "slime," or "log" the expression of perception accompanying atrocity. They are playing off a vision, the vision in Geller's "Why should it have a point? What point? It's just a physical system, what point is there?" They are playing with the line, as a gunner, perhaps, might play with a line of fire his shells make in a city.

In the principal documented instances of experimentation on human beings for the advancement of knowledge, with the human "material" being on the other side of the line, what was done was what might be done by anyone to dirt, log, or slime, or, in the European expression of the situation, vermin. When intelligently designed and carried out, the experiments on Jewish subjects in occupied Europe and on Chinese subjects in occupied China did produce useful knowledge about infection, frostbite, air pressure, and a number of other matters. We have noted the photos of the European experiments that may be watched on monitors in Washington. From Manchuria, a medical assistant reported that some time after being infected, a log who had been given a number[2] was tied down. "I cut him open from the chest to the stomach, and he screamed terribly, and his face was all twisted in agony. He made this unimaginable sound, he was screaming so horribly. But then finally he stopped. This was all in a day's work for the surgeons, but it really left an impression on me because it was my first time." He went on to explain the method of proceeding: "Vivisection should be done under normal circumstances. If we'd used anesthesia, that might have affected the body organs and blood vessels that we were examining. So we couldn't have used anesthetic."[3]

Frostbite research was routine, freezing proceeding until "arms, when struck with a short stick, emitted a sound resembling that which a board gives out when it is struck,"[4] and included experimentation on a three-day-old baby, temperature being measured with a needle stuck inside the infant's middle finger: "Usually a hand of a three-day-old infant is clenched into a fist . . . but by sticking the needle in, the middle finger could be kept straight to make the experiment easier."[5] For toxins, "prisoners under close guard were daily taken from the fourth floor to the third floor laboratories. . . . [T]hey were placed on beds, and told by the interpreter not to worry. The men in white gowns were doctors, the interpreter reassured them, and they were in Nanking to 'give you medicine to heal your bodies.' The victims were then quickly injected . . . and the doctors and technician then settled down to observe the subjects' reactions."[6]

If these things are not to be done, and are so terrible that we see the United States Environmental Protection Agency barring the use of human data from Nazi experiments,[7] and if there is a desire to integrate the human and the natural as we move forward in understanding, then a question, at the very least a question, is raised by accounts of (for instance) infection of chimpanzees that can be placed side by side with these mid-twentieth-century accounts of experimentation on numbered logs:

> Now, nearly 13 years after the first infection of a chimp with H.I.V., one has died and a few others are sick, apparently from AIDS. Jerom, a 13-year old male who was first infected in 1985, died early last year. . . . Another chimp . . . a male named Nathan, received a transfusion of Jerom's blood before the first ape's death. "We're certainly studying the effects on Nathan on a virological and immunological basis, and possibly looking at other chimps as well. . . . It's going to be interesting to look at what happened to Jerom and what's happening in Nathan and what possibly is happening in other chimps and try to correlate that with humans." H.I.V. isolated from Jerom's blood was introduced into two more chimpanzees three months ago, one by injection and the other by application to her cervix. . . . Two more chimps will be infected anally within the month. . . . The purpose of the experiment . . . is to develop a model of how H.I.V. is acquired through different mucous membranes.[8]

It was reported from Manchuria that all the subjects in one experiment "were forced to drink copious quantities of cholera-infected milk. The four that received no immunization contracted cholera and died. Several of those tested who received conventional cholera injections also became ill and died. The eight who were vaccinated with ultrasonic cholera vaccine showed no cholera symptoms."[9] If that report is of crime so terrible that it transcends the positive law of any nation, a war crime, a crime against humanity, and the line is moved, then a report on a surplus of chimpanzees becomes more problematical when it describes speculation about projects that might not be considered if biomedical chimps were scarce, including "a suggestion that a few chimps be fed meat tainted with mad cow disease, to see if they can become infected."[10] What seems so natural to say—"One thing about which practically all biomedical researchers agree, though, is that experiments on chimps will probably continue at some level. . . . '[W]e're going to need chimpanzees in the future'"[11]—will seem that much closer to the Manchurian bulletin board, on which was recorded every day data such as: "'Specific date; 3 *maruta*, numbers so and so, were given injections of so and so, x cc; we need x number of hearts, or x number of livers, etc.'"[12]

In fact, of course, the line of which we have spoken has always been a line of shades. Every act of kindness, every staying of the hand in general or in particular instances, indicates the shading of the line. One hears it said that we don't need more than system or process to "account" for animals and everything about them, or for human beings and everything about them. That is all one needs, or has, or is—all anything is. You might fear, for yourself, for others, and for the speaker, except that what we do reveals what we think, and what we actually think affects what we do. There are large pointers, such as the new constitutional protection of animals in Germany, the constitutional status of concern for animals in India and, now, a state of the United States, the federal Animal Welfare Act in the United States governing treatment of some animals in research as well as other contexts, the various crimes of cruelty to animals, the recent Treaty of Amsterdam adding a protocol to the constitution of the European Union "to ensure improved protection and respect for animals as sentient beings."[13] These are not statements of law imposed on experimental scientists as merely external constraints, to which they are unable to respond in good faith. Distinguished investigators, experimenting with the mechanisms of stress, limit themselves even in the degree and kind of stress they will induce. The question of affection in animals beyond their calculating intelligence or use of tools, or the question of animal consciousness, or of their own recognition of individuality, or of their aesthetic sense, are questions internal to professional science and less marginal at the end of the twentieth century than at its midpoint.[14]

But it is not the legal, the declarative, the academic that is so telling. It is the small gesture that opens belief to view and, as in the case of human vermin and human logs at mid-century, the response to the extreme. Two boys are burning a dog alive after pulling out its nails with pliers. The dog's cries fill the air. Can a passerby who opposes it and intervenes to stop it escape the implication of her own action that, for her, the dog is more than system, has some "spirit"— to use that litmus word? The boys burning their toy wooden dog would not pose such a problem for the passerby. The cry, without spirit, would be like the sound "ooh ooh" a car makes when brushed against if it is fitted with an alarm system to increase its survival chances.

Moreover, in intervening, perhaps with force, because she cannot not intervene (though she may say that the voice of the law prohibits the torture), she may well put her belief, along with the cry of the dog, beyond system. What she offers the boys, and us, by her action as well as her language, is what enters the opening in system and process. Torture has always posed the question of what is sometimes called an "objectivity" in morality. Torturing an animal does so too, but it does by virtue of the very association of torture with an animal. For her who sees a moral problem and would intervene, the spirit of an animal is not a cultural artifact present in some minds and not in others, in some lands and not in others. The animal does have spirit— or does not if the passerby is wholly untroubled by the two boys burning the living dog. And the boys? Their action speaks; but they may be troubled also, and in candor may say so, and say so in later gesture, of guilt or remorse, or of affection for another dog.

CONNECTION THROUGH SYSTEM

Standing back and looking at what we and others do, we can see the quivering of the line, the ambiguity in drawing it. We can also see the hesitations of the hand or stayings of the hand vary according to perceived similarity of system, pattern, process: from primates, to dogs, to other land mammals, with birds flying in the air and cetaceans swimming in the sea seeming to have their own places in our thought. But it is not similarity of system or connection through system that pushes the human, still viewed as human, into continuity with nature. Respect would not flow from similarity of system, any more than largeness or smallness of size, longness or shortness of time, flow from mere numerical difference. That I, as an individual, on my sole journey through the cosmos, have an inner mechanism that is similar to yours—no one suggests they are identical—is largely a matter of assumption and faith. As for you, if we met together you would know my language, my humor, my hopes and moods. You would know me. You would not know my mechanism, the inside of my head, the system there and in my body that accompanies what you see and hear and feel. Without opening me up and looking inside or introducing a deficit into me to see what happened, you must depend upon some little evidences, my bleeding, for example, which tells you that there is blood and a circulatory system, my temporary subsidence in what you suppose is sleep and my crying out in what you suppose is a dream. You would depend on these and the fact you have never seen or heard of the contrary—an utterly different system inside—when you or others have seen the human, rather like your assuming the earth is turning now from never having seen the contrary.

But compared with the number of times you have seen the sun, you will not have seen many systems inside a human being. You rely on the reports of others. They have seen only a few, and their reports are infused with their own faith. There are many sunrises, few examined mechanisms, and your reliance on reports at all is infused with faith in their good faith. You have moved back to a connection that precedes any matching of system.

And to much the same effect, the agony of race, in these last few centuries of what we think of as our own time, has been the overcoming of perceived *difference* in pattern and system, in nose and skin and hair, in blood and susceptibility to disease, to see the human nonetheless. Though slavery has not been confined to the physically different, physical difference has supported the owning, the breeding, the separation of mate from mate and child from parent, the pain and the killing—those things done to the song sparrow and not to the human child. Just within the human, and without regard to surrounding nature, animate or inanimate, it is spirit found the same that places an individual on the same side of the line with us, where, indeed, he can decline to have his particular mechanism inspected to determine whether it is similar despite apparent difference.

Sameness of spirit is a form of speaking and understanding, as opposed to "explanation," as we generally use the term, which blends into explaining away and putting behind us what nags at us. It may be inarticulate understanding and inarticulate speaking. Sameness of spirit is what individuals see and report in the opening in system and process, and what they see brings to them—even in and from landscape—the very forms and sounds of nature. The sameness with which a pushing of the line begins, and from which a particular interest in similarity of system or connection through system arises, is something of a unity. It is surely very different from the sameness of mechanisms, which remain quite separate, as any "particle" remains separate from another identical "particle" as long as in thought it remains a "particle." But there is also a difference, or, worse, a uniqueness, that is part of the other having spirit at all, the other whose presence makes you not alone and who, in speaking, is not yourself speaking to yourself (and for whom, for instance, you cannot consent).

CONNECTION BEYOND SYSTEM

This being so, this identity despite difference and not through similarity of system, it cannot be said just how far the line may be moved as we continue to talk and listen, even just to ourselves, any more than I, or you, can encompass what might enter once candor breaches total vision of the cosmos. Not to treat something other than human as a medium only, like a stone for our molding or a tool for our purposes, but (to any degree, however jerkily and inconsistently) as a source to be heard and, as we say, "learned" from, can *begin* with animals. It seems clear the learning from animals we do is not only of a practical kind. It can be more direct, from eye to eye, and can be learning how to be, for all purposes, rather than how to do, for some purpose. Vicki Hearne whom we have mentioned, J. M. Coetzee, Barbara Smuts are among those who have begun now to plumb and articulate this,[15] though long ago Meister Eckhart advised that "those who bring about wonderful things in their big, dark books take an animal to help them."[16] Such learning can continue where there is no physical sound to hear (except perhaps all sound) and no eye to look into (or to cover before we use or kill). There are many voices urging this further turn. Lewis Thomas's in *The Fragile Species* is I think one of them, for all his efforts to limit himself to an interest in the systems in which we find ourselves.

For Thomas, his speaking about the things of which he was speaking was not the clicking and rippling of systems; nor was our life, nor the larger life to which he wanted to introduce us, the co-alescence and dissolution of systems. We may start with recognizing, or hearing it urged that we recognize, the actuality in the other of love, or loyalty, or trust, or altruism, or a form of speech, or music or song, or courage, or humor, or play. But we do not end at the point where we can no longer easily speak in these terms of experience of the other, the sameness of the other, the other that makes us not alone, far though these terms—"love," "trust," and "play" especially—can take us without their losing all power to convey and evoke.

"Life" might be thought the more generic term and more widely acceptable than "spirit," the attempted exclusion of which—its negative mention is there—is a conventional mark of total theory. But "life" and "I live," or "it's alive," have rather parted company in our usage, and what makes "life" more acceptable than "spirit" is just that it has been shorn of that which raises a question where the line should be drawn, that which evokes the hesitant gesture, the wish the hand could be stayed. Worms live, and aerate the soil that sustains us. But it is generally only the child that swallows hard before he skewers the worm on a hook for the pleasure of catching a fish, pleasure which in this most complicated world may likely lead him as an adult to begin voicing claims of nature on humankind.

"Life" can nonetheless point to our thought and experience that is prior to our interest in system and process and not captured by them, and that can lead beyond system. There is active speculation on the presence of life elsewhere in the universe, and active search for it in the use of space probes, the search for planets around stars, the missions within our own solar system, and the listening for signals. What would satisfy the drive would not, I think, be discovery of a system that, like ours, is more or less self-replicating, or a system, also somewhat like ours, that seeks to use and organize what it (like us) might call the "materials" around it into patterns like its own—"materials" was the word used for human subjects in Manchuria when "logs" was not used. What would satisfy the drive would rather be the discovery that we are not alone.

And, to stay entirely within the experience of the human, the agonizing over when human life begins and when it ends—in others, of course, not ourselves except as life gains or loses meaning for us—is not helped by beginning with systems and excluding all else from discussion and reflection. When it is that this other is with us as a human being, and when no longer with us, are orphan questions, wandering intrusions on thought, when the eye is on systems. The eye ranges round, forming and reforming organizations of units for consideration, aspects coming into focus, fading, reappearing. Correlating with life or the human the presence or absence of one or another organization of units in a process, which we hold steady for a moment to see it with life or the human, is without guide, unless we have a guide from other experience. We argue over the placing of units into sets, though each set is as valid as any other until one is selected out for some purpose. But if the purpose is respect, treating the other as like ourselves, no set of units steps forward to say it should be the one.

The pulmonary and circulatory system is a unit and part of the great atmospheric balancing of O_2 and CO_2, as is a tree, if you stand back and view a tree as such. The stomach is part of the agricultural system, through which the agricultural system's products flow; and a stomach, joining other stomachs, is part of the sewerage and recycling systems, that receive the processed agricultural product. As the eye ranges, seeing now this connection and now that, each system of a human being, each "part," is seen as part of many systems. Is one part or one arrangement necessary to life or the human? When thinking exclusively of systems, even our special concern for the presence of a brain may be viewed as "privileging" it, for reasons of "culture" that are in fact the operative units and forces of just another system. We could "privilege" the stomach, as in the imagery of Homer or as we do with the fixed sea-dwelling molluscs filtering plankton, any one of which without a stomach would hardly *be* one of its kind.

Discussion of life and the human, and discussion of systems, are not the same; and though we must and do agonize, and must and do make decisions, we cannot stop the agonizing by saying simply that we choose to attribute life to one or another of the various ways of looking at the organization of units, and choose to make one or another feature crucial, in pursuit of our purposes. For the distinctive feature of life and the human (in its recognition by us) is that it is not entirely subject to our purposes. Discussions of when transitional forms of hominids have reached the human, or whether the Neanderthal, if independently evolved, was human, seem restless, rootless, looking now at cranial capacity, now at tool use, now at genetic structure. Afflicting such discussion is the same arbitrariness afflicting discussions confined to the presence and functioning of systems and seeking to establish when in an individual life the human is there, and when it is no longer present.

Indeed in the judgments about the human in evolution, which have to do with our more general sense of ourselves, the evidence of prehistoric art may be more important to us than we know. Or the evidence of mourning and burial—but then elephants may mourn and cover their dead.

Justification and Compensation

The shading already seen in the line, and the recognition and identification that may come, do not mean that experimental science will ultimately be impossible to carry out or that medical advance will stop. We are in systems. We are in competition, with each other and with that which is not human. Economists do have a subject. There is scarcity, and not just of time available to understand the nature of the world from our own work and experience and the work and experience reported by others.

Among the systems in which we find ourselves situated is the system of nutrition, which though it is as domestic and familiar as the kitchen may be as difficult to fathom as the system of criminal justice—fathom not in the sense of understanding "how" but in the sense of understanding "why," the "why" that cannot be wholly folded into the "how." Fathoming it includes, where our action is concerned, justifying to ourselves what we do.

The mutuality of dependence of systems does not alchemically lead to respect and forbearance. The farmer is dependent upon his rich plot of earth for his own sustenance, the plot of earth is dependent for its richness upon what the farmer does for it. But the line of which we have spoken does not, for that reason alone, enter the farmer's consideration, or ours.

And the contrary, the failure of mutual dependency, does not lead to the utter absence of respect and forbearance. Backed into a corner you destroy what would destroy you, your enemy, but there are ways of destruction that acknowledge the line, the presence before you, and your connection. You may bury his body with care. Wilderness may threaten, and care or liking for us may be nowhere in it; but for those who see value in it this is of no consequence—if they are not backed into a corner, and, for some, even if they are.

Our attitude toward the animal part of nature that is not human, and that feeds human beings (and if not eaten must be fed), is so nicely reflected in the story of the pig with the wooden leg that we might let it take us lightly toward our parting.

A man was walking down a country road and saw over the fence a pig with a wooden leg. A bit further along he came upon the farmer.

"Could I ask you why that pig has a wooden leg?"

"That pig!" the farmer said. "Let me tell you about that pig. That's a most extraordinary pig. Not long ago I was plowing on my tractor and it turned over, pinning my leg. The tractor was sinking into the mud and would have crushed it. That pig rushed over, smashed through the fence, wedged his body under the tractor tire and held it up. I owe this leg to that pig."

"Yes," the traveler replied, "that is most remarkable. I see your leg is fine. But I don't understand why the pig has a wooden leg."

"Let me tell you something else about that pig," said the farmer. "Just last week my family and I were asleep upstairs in our house over there. A fire broke out in the kitchen in the middle of the night and the house filled with smoke. The pig saw it, broke through the fence again, pushed open the door and rushed upstairs and pulled us out of bed. My whole family owes its life to that pig."

"Yes, I see," said the visitor. "But you still haven't told me why it has a wooden leg."

"Oh," the farmer said. "Well, a pig like that, you wouldn't want to eat it all at once."

Dependence does not stop use. The emphasis cannot be upon dependence, but upon the qualities that blur the line and raise the question of justification—here the pig's altruism and devotion. Eating slowly does not seem quite the response, a wooden leg quite enough compensation.

Recognition, in a setting of necessity. Though it be attended by evasion, recognition takes us into a world of justification and compensation that we may not have been in before and, at its extreme, a world of limits, of agony and forbearance, that were not present before. "Remorse," "penance," "paying," the old words, the words indeed of criminal law, become pertinent even to scientific work. So much of inquiry in the criminal law is into whether the one who has hurt or destroyed was doing the best he could in good faith. Recognition does not mean no animal can be sacrificed, but, with recognition, use must be seen as sacrifice, in an older sense than the word is now used in the laboratory. Struggle within ourselves need not always lead to forbearance, nor death or deprivation at our hand be always condemned, but there must be struggle.

THE CONVERGENCE OF SCIENTIFIC AND OTHER FORMS OF THOUGHT

Over time and in the large, the presence of struggle, demand for justification, and possibility of limits will have an effect. Though blurring or moving the line does not mean an end to experiment or medical advance—after all, we hurt and kill one another in war, and through law, and by conscious neglect—it does mean that certain kinds of knowledge may be more difficult to have, and the sources and methods of achieving knowledge may tend to resemble one another more.

Predictive and manipulative knowledge, essential to our well-being, is not knowledge of things central to our being, love or loyalty, or meaning. There is always an effort to absorb the second knowledge into the first: partly, as we can see again and again, to escape responsibility, partly simply as a consequence of the division of our situation. If there is an other, and the other is thought about and acted upon differently, there is a pull to absorb us into the other—the schoolchild in us will recall osmosis at a membrane.

Our concern now is the reverse, the pulling of the other into us, and the consequences of thinking about it and acting upon it in something of the same way as we think about and want and try to act upon ourselves.

To predict love, manipulate loyalty, is to destroy them. To capture them and press them into units, and attach them, as units, to systems and make them part of systems is to destroy them. The same is true of the musical in music. It is the very point made in visual art. Craft is so critically important, but most critical is knowing that craft is not enough. Knowledge of love, loyalty, humor, courage, song, life, death—a voice here and a voice there adding words—is not of the predictive and manipulative kind.

There may be a fear such knowledge will be affected by a blurring or movement of the line, that with our increased sensitivity to systems within us and in which we live, and with our success in manipulating systems, the very knowing of these things may fade. But that it need not fade has been the point of our close reading here of what might initially seem threatening visions, threatening urgings and arguments. It is one thing to borrow and project words onto systems (or what are designated as systems), "community," for instance, as in a "community of trees," or "messages," with which hormones are said to work, or the "needs" of a nutritional system. It is another thing to believe. There is manipulation, combination, deprivation, elimination, and rearrangement of these systems, and discussion of the results, in these terms, "communicating," "acting in tandem," "satisfying needs," "dying." And then there is, to be sure, a turning back to discuss our community and our speaking and our needs in the same way. But that is just talk, open to interpretation and an asking for candor. Belief is what attaches words to reality; and it is up to the listener to determine whether belief is there, and it is the listener who can help the speaker see whether belief is there.

When we sense or see community, messages, or needs, or loyalty, love, song, courage, or humor *actually* in the other, our action comes into question. Things we *do* to the other as system only, that we do to the other because it is the other, would be a great crime if we were to do the same where we are concerned. Then "as if" stops. Then the return from the other to us is not just talk. What is done to the other might be done to us. What is done in pursuit of knowledge of a predictive and manipulative kind about these very things that are central to our being can destroy them in their actuality. Here moving the line will begin to show its first consequence. As the line between us and the other is blurred, action against the other may be stayed lest the same happen to us. Even discussion of these things central to our being in terms of system and process, prediction and manipulation, may be heard less. Listening to the song of the song sparrow as a song, not a "song" that is an arrangement of sounds produced by a system, may in fact help us listen to our own song.

Hearing the cry of the dog as a cry may help us hear the cry of a human being as a cry, and help us act in response to it.

With regard to knowledge that *is* of systems, the question of consent enters as the line moves, and with it the thrust of the Nuremberg Code on experimentation without consent.[17] Between human being and human being, the question of consent is vexed enough. Even agreeing on when true consent is assured has been difficult, what degree of disclosure, understanding, and freedom from duress are necessary to it, and how usefully one can think about quantified risks on one's own behalf.[18] It is urged that no prisoner and no one in financial need can be viewed as truly consenting, even that no one but the experimenter himself has sufficient knowledge and understanding to consent to experimentation in many cases, which would make himself the only available subject for experimentation. With the other than human, there may be no possibility of consent. If the concerns remain the same as within the human, the impossibility of consent will not mean it is irrelevant: the child can no more give consent than the song sparrow.

But the question of consent is only an aspect of the general problem of justification. If individuality is seen in the other, so that the question of death, that we face, is faced there, if some degree of consciousness is seen there so that the fear of death enters, then "sacrifice" in experimentation becomes sacrifice as of old with all that means and entails. Again, this only enhances the degree of justification that we may ask of ourselves or others, which rises or falls with the degree of suffering, in ourselves or others, and with which the degree of compensation of one kind or another rises and falls. There may be no absolute bar. But knowledge gained through the techniques of experimentation, through separation and combination, rearrangement, and introduction of deficits including the ultimate deficit which is death, may not be had so freely. It may be gained once, but not often again, it may be gained once and never again: if built on the back of death and violation, as was the knowledge obtained in German or Manchurian death camps about how much pressure the human body could bear or how fast the human body uses up its last resources of its own fat for nourishment, it may simply be no longer available through replication of experiment.

Thus as the line moves or is blurred in our sight, confirmation of knowledge—generation by generation—may no longer be fully available or available for all, all including each individual one of us appearing new in the world wanting to know of the world, and then to have what is said to be known of it demonstrated, to see it with one's own eyes.

The one special claim to truth that is made for scientific truth about the systems and processes of the world is that it can be demonstrated, that there need be no dependence on the good faith of others or deference to the authority of others, that anyone on earth, given enough capacity of mind, time, and resources, can see the truth for himself or herself. It is this that undergirds scientific belief about things and distinguishes scientific belief as different. We return to our starting point, that truth believed to be truth, and action, are connected. They are connected in the way we have discussed here, in legal method and in life. They are connected in their own way in the scientific endeavor.

The ways of connection have never been entirely different. Though good faith and trust cannot be much defined or much manipulated, the sense of them and of their reality may come from an equally clear-eyed attention to what works, in keeping a society together, or keeping a life going. The passion for the empirical there is in science may be no less in that which is not science. Resources, time, variation in capacity and focus may already make constant replication impossible, and movement of the line may be thought to make practical impossibility only that much more so in degree.

But the consequence over time may be a convergence of the scientific form of thought and other forms of thought, and a merging of scientific truth and other truth. With necessity, that blocks seeing for oneself, being not an external constraint one can imagine getting around but a necessity of justification, with the hand stayed not by time or resources or the distribution of individual capacities but by identification with that which the hand might have seized, the distinctiveness of scientific method will be less and less easily seen, and the source of scientific knowledge, from generation to generation, will no longer be so different from other sources of knowledge.

The good faith of others reporting will become the more important if one cannot see for oneself. The interpretation of others' speech will be the more important as Nature cannot be forced to speak. The close reading of a person may be as common in science as in law. The metaphorical and the mathematical will both be avenues to insight and understanding. Science and what is not science—there would be no antiscience—will both proceed on premises and faiths that come from a world that is more than a world of system and process. They may find a meeting place in law. Scientists and those who do not devote their lives to science must meet there in any event, to trace the line of action and suffering and decide where the sparrow is to be put, and the child.

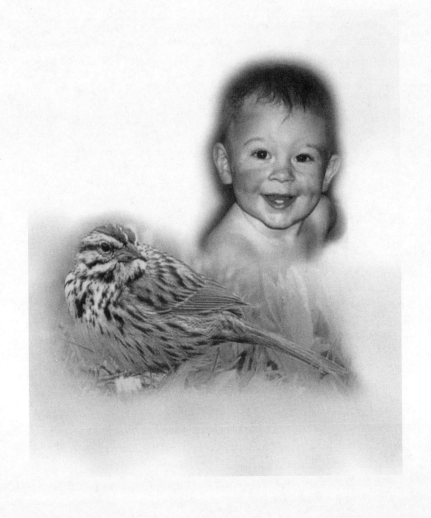

Notes

INTRODUCTION

1. William James, *Pragmatism* (Cambridge, MA: Harvard University Press, 1975) (first published 1907), 9, quoting G. K. Chesterton.

Chapter 1.   THE SONG SPARROW AND THE CHILD

1. Lewis Thomas, *The Fragile Species* (New York: Macmillan, 1992), 160, 24.
2. Nicholas D. Kristof, "Japan Confronting Gruesome War Atrocity," *New York Times*, March 17, 1995.
3. Christian Pross and Götz Aly, *The Value of the Human Being: Medicine in Germany, 1918–1945* (Berlin: Ärztekammer Berlin, 1991), 15, 22, 38.
4. John R. Searle, *The Rediscovery of the Mind* (Cambridge, MA: MIT Press, 1992), 89–90; *The Construction of Social Reality* (New York: The Free Press, 1995), xi–xii; *Rediscovery*, 86–87.
5. J. J. C. Smart, "Professor Ziff on Robots," in *Minds and Machines: Contemporary Perspectives in Philosophy Series,* ed. Alan Ross Anderson (Englewood Cliffs, NJ: Prentice-Hall, 1964), 105.
6. Murray Gell-Mann, *The Quark and the Jaguar: Adventures in the Simple and the Complex* (New York: W. H. Freeman, 1994), 33.
7. François Jacob, *The Logic of Life: A History of Heredity* and *The Possible and the Actual,* trans. Betty S. Spillmann (London: Penguin, 1982), 2, 307, 245, 299, 248, 421, 306.
8. Sheldon H. Harris, *Factories of Death: Japanese Biological Warfare, 1932–1945, and the American Cover-Up* (London: Routledge, 1994), 49, 62.
9. David Chandler, *Voices from S-21: Terror and History in Pol Pot's Secret Prison* (Berkeley: University of California Press, 1999), 143, 147, 150–53.

10. Jean-Pierre Changeux and Alain Connes, *Conversations on Mind, Matter, and Mathematics,* ed. and trans. M. B. DeBevoise (Princeton: Princeton University Press, 1995), 26, 38.

11. Steven Weinberg, *The First Three Minutes: A Modern View of the Origin of the Universe* (1977) (New York: Basic Books, 1993), 154.

12. Steven Weinberg, *Dreams of a Final Theory* (New York: Pantheon Books, 1992), 255.

13. Stephen W. Hawking, *A Brief History of Time: From the Big Bang to Black Holes,* with an introduction by Carl Sagan (New York: Bantam Books, 1988), 174–75.

14. "Unreasonable effectiveness" is Eugene Wigner's often quoted phrase. See Changeux and Connes, *Conversations,* xi, 47, 51, 422.

Chapter 2. THE CLOSE READING OF COSMOLOGIES

1. Lewis Thomas, *The Lives of a Cell: Notes of a Biology Watcher* (New York: Bantam Books, 1974).

2. Lewis Thomas, *The Medusa and the Snail: More Notes of a Biology Watcher* (New York: Bantam Books, 1980).

3. Lewis Thomas, *Late Night Thoughts on Listening to Mahler's Ninth Symphony* (New York: Viking, 1983). A Lewis Thomas Scientist as Poet Prize has been established by Rockefeller University.

4. Thomas, *Fragile Species.* Lewis Thomas died December 3, 1993.

5. Jacques Monod, *Chance and Necessity: An Essay on the Natural Philosophy of Modern Biology,* trans. Austryn Wainhouse (New York: Alfred A. Knopf, 1971), 172.

6. Weinberg, *Dreams of a Final Theory.*

7. Betty Jo Teeter Dobbs, *The Janus Faces of Genius: The Role of Alchemy in Newton's Thought* (Cambridge: Cambridge University Press, 1991). See also, on the history of chemistry, Roald Hoffman, *The Same and Not the Same* (New York: Columbia University Press, 1995).

8. John Maynard Keynes, *Essays in Biography,* ed. Geoffrey Keynes (New York: W. W. Norton, 1963), 310–23; Richard H. Popkin, *The Third Force in Seventeenth Century Thought* (Leiden: E. J. Brill, 1992), 172–202; Richard S. Westfall, *The Life of Isaac Newton* (Cambridge: Cambridge University Press, 1993).

9. Lewis Thomas, "Introduction," in H. F. Judson, *The Search for Solutions* (New York: Holt, Rinehart and Winston, 1980), x.

10. In speaking of language itself as a "property" Thomas uses a language of "property" or "properties" that has a legal ring to it—"that is mine, my property." Its use especially indicates control over the subject of discourse. But what human language cannot do, above all, is seize and fix a human experience apart from the speaker and listener. There is something of the young love of magic displayed in the widespread convention of proceeding by "definition," something of the shaman in us all because we all do it. No discourse—except perhaps poetry—is exempt from the temptation to believe that if something has been put into a word or words, especially the words of a definition, it is captured, it stays.

There is seduction, to be sure, in law's language of "property." The word signals a move into the world of ownership and into a particular form of legal analysis, basic and important. Economic and commercial thought and activity depend upon it and, some would say, even recognition of the human individual. What any transferred use of law's word "property" leaves behind, forgets or must forget, is that in the world of "ownership" each exclusion, each taking, each holding on, each order enforced on the basis of a claim to exclude or take or hold, is if challenged a consequence of a responsible decision after argument.

Mathematicians also speak of a "property," and perhaps the tendency to call mathematics a "language" obscures what human language cannot do to or for human experience. The tendency, an old one, is particularly pronounced at the beginning of the twentieth-first century. Mathematics is often called not just a language, but the one universal language. Those who say this of mathematics move away from human language, to avoid the personal, and to have a universal language. They may actually say this is the language of heaven, like Sanskrit, Hebrew, or Arabic before, with an existence independent of those who work with it.

The *desire* is to grasp and hold. The "idea of science" is a "property," in Jacques Monod's parallel evolution of the system of human culture (*Chance and Necessity*, 165, 170). The "concept of liberty" is a "property," in Changeux's and Connes's arguments over the working of the human mind (*Conversations*, 29–30). If one can perfect (the legal term) a claim of property, one can not only grasp and hold. One can escape for a moment the terrible question of purpose and judgment of purpose: one can "do what one wants with one's own," boxed as it is within its defining walls. Lawyers and judges in practice see so much of the desire and the claim. They know the relief given by the escape from purpose that "property" brings, perhaps the necessity of some such relief, as they work constantly with what is to be a "property" or analyzed as such, and what is not. But lawyer and judge as well as citizen juror know that a claim of property cannot be perfected on all the world.

11. Jonathan Sacks, *Faith in the Future* (London: Darton, Longman and Todd, 1995), 49, 86.

12. Rilke, who spent much time in the Paris Zoo, had written in the *Duino Elegies* (which must have been known to Thomas), "The shrewd animals / notice that we're not very much at home / in the world we've expounded." Rainer Maria Rilke, *Duino Elegies,* trans. C. F. MacIntyre (Berkeley: University of California Press, 1961).

13. Hawking, *Brief History of Time,* 152–53.

Chapter 3.   EVERYTHING, ONLY, AND NOTHING BUT

1. Searle, *Rediscovery,* 85–86, 89–91.

2. *The Brain,* Proceedings of the American Academy of Arts and Sciences, *Daedalus,* vol. 127, no. 2 (Spring 1998).

3. Oliver Sacks, *An Anthropologist on Mars* (New York: Vintage Books, 1995), 298, 5–6, 99.

4. Steven Rose, "Beyond the Gene's-Eye View," *Times Literary Supplement,* March 13, 1998, 12.

5. Semir Zeki, "Art and the Brain," in *The Brain,* 99; see also Zeki, *Inner Vision: An Exploration of Art and the Brain* (Oxford: Oxford University Press, 1999), 1. "Rules" that all human activities "must obey": metaphorical the language may be, but this metaphor is especially legal, and it has a familiar echo. "Rules, must obey" is not a reference to authority that evokes the internalization of joint purpose. The authoritarian and its difference from the authoritative come immediately to mind—the scientist saying "must obey" knows it like any other human being. Oscillation between the search for the authoritative and the fall into the authoritarian is part of ordinary life, and law especially struggles with it within itself.

6. "Joseph Weizenbaum: 'The Myth of the Last Metaphor,'" in Peter Baumgartner and Sabine Payr, eds., *Speaking Minds: Interviews with Twenty Eminent Cognitive Scientists* (Princeton: Princeton University Press, 1995), 249–64. Weizenbaum's DOCTOR, a psychoanalytic script using his language analysis program ELIZA and written as a spoof, attracted so much serious attention that he withdrew for two years from his work in computer programming to write his general testament, *Computer Power and Human Reason: From Judgment to Calculation* (New York: W. H. Freeman, 1976).

7. Bruno Bettelheim, *Freud and Man's Soul* (New York: Vintage Books, 1984).

8. See Edward T. Linenthal, *Preserving Memory: The Struggle to Create America's Holocaust Museum* (New York: Viking, 1995), 196; United States Holocaust Museum, 2002, ushmm.org/research/collections, "Film and Video," "Museum's Permanent Exhibition," "The Holocaust: View photographs of this exhibition from the Photo Archives," #49, Photograph NO3889.20, "Visitors view the medical experiment monitors on the third floor of the permanent exhibition in the United States Holocaust Museum."

9. Baumgartner and Payr, *Speaking Minds,* 256−60. Compare the opening statement of the prosecutor Telford Taylor at the Nuremberg Trial of experimenters on concentration camp inmates: "To their murderers, these wretched people were not individuals at all. They came in wholesale lots and were treated worse than animals. . . . The defendants in the dock are charged with murder, but this is no mere murder trial. . . . These defendants did not kill in hot blood, nor for personal enrichment. . . . They are not ignorant men. Most of them are trained physicians and some of them are distinguished scientists. . . . It is our deep obligation to all peoples of the world to show why and how these things happened . . . the ideas and motives which moved these defendants to treat their follow men as less than beasts." *Trials of War Criminals Before the Nuernberg Military Tribunals Under Control Council Law No. 10, October 1946−April 1949,* "The Medical Case," vol. 1, 27−28 (U.S. Government Printing Office). The connection in this passage between thinking (or not thinking) of "murder" and perceiving an "individual" is common, and, indeed, ultimately affects the treatment of animals also.

10. Jacob, *The Logic of Life,* 322.

11. See Frans de Waal, *Good Natured: The Origins of Right and Wrong in Humans and Other Animals* (Cambridge, MA: Harvard University Press, 1996), 226 n. 12. Compare "attachment" experiments on rhesus monkeys, involving maternal deprivation and social isolation, described in Deborah Blum, *Love at Goon Park: Harry Harlow and the Science of Affection* (New York: Perseus, 2002), e.g., 203−25.

Chapter 4. IDENTIFYING SCIENCE

1. Thomas, "Introduction," *Search for Solutions,* x.

2. See also Michael Redhead, "Other Universes," reviewing David Deutsch's *The Fabric of Reality* and Lee Smolin's *The Life of the Cosmos,*

Times Literary Supplement, January 2, 1998, 5. It has been important to some recently to argue that evolution is without direction—toward "complexity" (if "complexity" can ever be defined excluding human interest), or away from it. See, e.g., Stephen Jay Gould, *Full House: The Spread of Excellence from Plato to Darwin* (New York: Random House, 1997). Compare Simon Conway Morris, *Life's Solution: Inevitable Humans in a Lonely Universe* (Cambridge: Cambridge University Press, 2003); Morris, "Where Are We Headed?" reviewing Robert Wright's *Nonzero, New York Times Book Review,* January 30, 2000, 6; Freeman Dyson, *Imagined Worlds* (Cambridge, MA: Harvard University Press, 1997). Where total theory is presented in the language of "emergent properties" it varies of course with the person presenting it. "Emergence" as generally described is offered to replace a "determinism" that is not thought to acknowledge adequately the presence of chance or the importance of evolution. In addition to Changeux and Connes, *Conversations,* contemporary summaries of "emergence" can be found in the computer scientist John H. Holland's *Emergence: From Chaos to Order* (Reading, MA: Addison-Wesley, 1998) and the physicist and Nobelist Murray Gell-Mann's *The Quark and the Jaguar: Adventures in the Simple and the Complex.* A brief but particularly sensitive exploration can be found in the physicist Sir Brian Pippard's "Master-Minding the Universe," *Times Literary Supplement,* July 29, 1983, 795–96. Raymond Tallis's *Psycho-Electronics* (London: Ferrington, 1994) is a brief and readable critical analysis of many of the theoretical terms.

The contribution legal thought can make to other disciplines considering these matters, and to the general reader doing so, is to recall and point to individual and person as elemental—in a daily way to remind all of us talking about the nature of things that it is *we* who are talking.

Indeed, human language in which law lives has its own way of taking care of the grasp at everything. When all human experience is pressed into "properties," for insertion into systems and processes that would fill the world, the speaker and the listener reappear. Try letting a total theory of emergent properties exist on its own. Put it into a box, as a discrete idea, a concept, a definition, and set it out. Start, for example, with the phrase, "All is process." This is "historicism"—total theory is found not just in the talk of physicists, biologists, or mathematicians. All is a contingency, thrown up by process, removed by process—all is history. Is historicism too a contingency thrown up by process? It would seem so. That it is a flash of insight into objective truth cannot be allowed. "All is process" must be swallowed into . . . what? Not *process.* The very idea, "process," is contingent and must pass. Pass into what then? Darkness? Whose darkness? Ours—

we are here. And do we who are here know nothing, are we wholly in dark ignorance? No. We know we are here speaking, as we also know that we are in systems and processes. If I stood before you and said, "all is process," in that word "all," if you took me to mean "all" as I usually mean all and you usually mean all, I will have said—or seemed to have said—that I know nothing. And the question is put for you, and then for me, What am I actually saying, standing there, speaking to you?

Similarly, evolution on its own terms, if expressed as a theory of everything, is an emergent property that will survive or not—in itself as something discrete, and as part of a system of other emergent properties—depending upon its relative advantage against competitors in whatever environment faces them all in the future (an environment that is, of course, a system, to which they themselves contribute). At the point where evolutionary theory becomes a total theory, a vision of all aspects of the organic and perhaps the very laws of physics themselves as units combining and recombining in systems and systems of systems by variation and selection, theory itself must necessarily become a "natural phenomenon." Theory too, by definition, must become a combination of units, a system, a system of systems, a property of a system of systems. It is not different in kind from "anger" or "love," "human law" or "the human mind," "responsibility" or "remorse," "forgiveness" or "horror," which by definition must be combinations of units, systems, systems of systems, properties of systems.

The theory of evolution *was,* on its own terms, a chance variation, selected, for this moment, to survive. It and a system of which it becomes a part *will,* through a "diversity generator" (such as the behavior of material in DNA) produce further emergent properties, which will themselves form a system that may or may not be selected further for survival. But it, the theory, and the system of which it becomes a part, will produce further emergent properties that may be so selected, only if it and its system happen to survive to do so, against other systems producing properties in the same way. There is not truth in what the system which is the tongue, the hand, or the eye registers in sound or script from the system which is the mind or brain. There is only, in the theory's world that includes the theory, chance variation, systemization, and selection, in competition with other sequences of chance variation, systemization, and selection going on all around it. *It,* on its own terms, this very vision of chance variation, systemization, and selection with no assurance of survival, is as divorced from a true view of the world as much as any other chance variation. It once was not, is now, may not be for long— that is all that can be said, and really not even that, if the terms of the vision extend to everything, if it is accompanied by phrases such as "all," "entire," "whole," "only," "nothing but." Connes, the mathematician, perceives this vanishing, this endpoint of radical ignorance, and, speaking for himself and for other mathematicians, rejects it, for mathematics.

In seeing circular swallowing when a system which is total is packaged, presented, and urged, it may be thought one is seeing a "problem of logic." It is not a "problem of logic" that is actually seen. These urgings of total visions point so nicely beyond themselves, to where, standing outside the talk, are the persons talking.

The most sensitive and engaging treatment of self-obliteration in epistemology, and its history, is to be found in George Levine's *Dying to Know* (Chicago: University of Chicago Press, 2002), see, e.g., 85–103, 268–83. See also his *Darwin and the Novelists* (Cambridge, MA: Harvard University Press, 1988; Chicago: University of Chicago Press, 1991), 235–37, 271–72.

3. Searle, *Construction,* 120.

4. Peter Davison, *The Fading Smile: Poets in Boston, from Robert Frost to Robert Lowell to Sylvia Plath, 1955–1960* (New York: Alfred A. Knopf, 1994).

Chapter 5. THE PROBLEM OF THE NEGATIVE

1. See Clifford Geertz, "Life Among the Anthros," *New York Review of Books,* February 8, 2001, 18–22, and the references therein; American Anthropological Association, *El Dorado Task Force Final Report,* vols. I & II, May 18, 2002. Did Neel have a totalizing vision in which there were no real lines for action to cross, or not to cross? For readers of his autobiography he may have made an effort to close the opening here in the systems with which he worked, by making "epiphanic experience" an "attribute." *Physician to the Gene Pool* (New York: John Wiley & Sons, 1994), 189. We should have to read his active life and listen closely to his entire testimony to judge.

2. William H. Calvin, *How Brains Think: Evolving Intelligence, Then and Now* (New York: Basic Books, 1996), 148–49.

3. Marcea Bartusiak, "The Mechanics of the Soul: A Prominent Neurophysiologist Argues That Consciousness Is the Result of Evolution," *New York Times Book Review,* November 17, 1996.

4. Brian Rotman, *Ad Infinitum: The Ghost in Turing's Machine* (Stanford: Stanford University Press, 1993).

5. Ian Kershaw, *Hitler 1936–1945: Nemesis* (New York: W. W. Norton, 2000), 130, 424–26, 428; "Dabru Emet: A Jewish Statement on Christians and Christianity," National Jewish Scholars Project, 2000; Office of Strategic Services Research and Analysis Branch, July 6, 1945, "The Persecution of

the Christian Churches," *Rutgers Journal of Law & Religion,* www-camlaw. rutgers.edu/publications/law-religion/.

6. See George J. Annas and Michael A. Grodin, eds., *The Nazi Doctors and the Nuremberg Code: Human Rights in Human Experimentation* (New York: Oxford University Press, 1992); Linenthal, *Preserving Memory,* 196.

7. *Unnecessary Fuss,* narrated by Ingrid Newkirk and compiled by Alex Pacheco, excerpts from videotapes from the University of Pennsylvania Head Injury Clinic (Washington, DC: People for the Ethical Treatment of Animals, Inc., 1985).

8. See, e.g., Hans Moravec, *Mind Children: The Future of Robot and Human Intelligence* (Cambridge, MA: Harvard University Press, 1988), 65–74; Douglas R. Hofstadter, *Le Ton beau de Marot: In Praise of the Music of Language* (New York: Basic Books, 1997), 488–93; Ray Kurzweil, *The Age of Spiritual Machines: When Computers Exceed Human Intelligence* (New York: Penguin, 2000), 261–80.

9. Baumgartner and Payr, *Speaking Minds,* 257–58.

10. Arthur Koestler, *Darkness at Noon* (New York: Bantam Books, 1968) (first published 1941).

11. Ute Deichmann, *Biologists under Hitler,* trans. Thomas Dunlap (Cambridge, MA: Harvard University Press, 1996), 398 n. 47.

12. Elias Canetti, *Crowds and Power,* trans. Carol Stewart (New York: Farrar, Straus and Giroux, 1984). The gestalt psychologist Wolfgang Köhler, widely known for *The Mentality of Apes* (1917), set out a total theory that was to identify "modern science in general" in his 1934 William James Lectures, *The Place of Value in a World of Facts* (New York: Liveright, 1938); see chapter 10, "Man and Nature," 390–94. Köhler acknowledged and confronted— in a particularly explicit way—absorption of theorist into theory when ultimately the explainer is explained as a system: "[T]he human organism represents a physical system all the characteristics of which will sooner or later be traced to the constituents and to the fundamental laws of nature in general. . . . [W]e shall deny that life is governed by any principles which are as such essentially different from those of the inorganic world. . . . The very being that observes physical facts in the narrower sense of the word, that thinks about these facts, and that thus builds up the science of physics, constitutes at the same time the most challenging subject-matter of that discipline. . . . [A]ny characteristics of man that are involved in the creation of physics will fall under the same rule."

The institutional vision of a major American research university at the end of the twentieth century may be compared: "The field of life sciences holds extraordinary promise for the next century as it continues to push the

frontiers of knowledge about every aspect of biological life. . . . Closely allied to the life sciences are the social sciences, which, though distinctive in
their definition, are in fact concerned with a particular level of analysis of
living organisms (usually humans). Indeed, the boundaries between neuroscience (a life science) and psychology (a social science) are rather indistinct and are becoming increasingly more so. . . . [T]he laws of physics and
chemistry should, in principle, be able to explain and predict biological
phenomena in a precise manner. Understanding these aspects of the life
sciences in the terms of mathematical modeling and theoretical applica-
tions of universal laws and principles is one of our greatest challenges for
the next century." *Report of the President's Commission on the Life Sciences,
University of Michigan, 1999,* ix, 5, 61.

13. See Erich Fromm, *Marx's Concept of Man* (New York: Frederick
Ungar, 1961).

14. Robert D. Kaplan, *Balkan Ghosts: A Journey through History* (New
York: St. Martin's Press, 1993), xviii, 95.

Chapter 7. WAYS OF KNOWING AND THE QUESTION
OF SCIENTIFIC METHOD

1. G.H. Hardy, *A Mathematician's Apology,* with a foreword by C.P.
Snow (Cambridge: Cambridge University Press, 1982) (first published
1940), 127–28.

2. Nicolas Wade, "Doctors Question Use of Nazis' Medical Atlas,"
New York Times, November 26, 1996; Marjorie Sun, "EPA Bars Use of Nazi
Data," *Science,* vol. 240, 21; Jay Katz and Robert S. Pozos, "The Dachau Hy-
pothermia Study, An Ethical and Scientific Commentary," and Jay Katz,
"Abuse of Human Beings for the Sake of Science," in Arthur L. Caplan,
ed., *When Medicine Went Mad: Bioethics and the Holocaust* (Totawa, NJ:
Humana Press, 1992), 135, 263. See also Steven Dickman, "Memorial Cere-
mony to Be Held," *Nature,* vol. 345 (1990), 192 (on the 1990 burial of brains
collected from extermination center inmates for study). In World War II
experiments on Chinese, "Still others brought to their work a dedication
derived from a belief that working on human subjects was no different
than doing research with plant or animal specimens. . . . Unit 100 . . . 'in-
vestigated the action of bacteria by means of experiments on domestic
animals and human beings, for which purpose the detachment had horses,
cows and other animals, and also kept human beings in isolation cells.' . . .
[It] was composed essentially of bacteriologists, chemists, veterinarians, and

agronomists. . . . After completing a brief mission to Japan in November 1947, Edwin V. Hill, M.D., Chief, Basic Sciences, Camp Detrick, Maryland, observed, 'Evidence gathered in this investigation has greatly supplemented and amplified previous aspects of this field.' The data gathered by enemy scientists was secured 'at the expenditure of many millions of dollars and years of work. . . . Such information could not be obtained in our own laboratories because of scruples attached to human experimentation.'" Harris, *Factories*, 44, 91, 66. The well-known Milgram experiments, demonstrating the lengths human subjects would go, in deference to the orders of scientific investigators, to harm or kill others whom they were tricked to believe were actually being harmed, are an example of what might not be repeatable in the behavioral sciences as informed consent becomes more widely required. See Ruth R. Faden and Tom L. Beauchamp, *The History and Theory of Informed Consent* (New York: Oxford University Press, 1986).

3. E.g., Herbert A. Simon, *The Sciences of the Artificial,* 2d ed. (Cambridge, MA: MIT Press, 1981), 64–66.

Chapter 8.   THE OPENING AND THE LINE

1. Vicki Hearne, *Adam's Task: Calling Animals by Name* (New York: Alfred A. Knopf, 1986).

2. Weinberg, *Dreams of a Final Theory,* 242.

3. Monod, *Chance and Necessity,* 171–72.

4. *Rome* (Clermont-Ferrand: Michelin et Cie, 2002), 310.

5. Lon L. Fuller, *The Morality of Law* (New Haven: Yale University Press, 1969); *The Law in Quest of Itself* (Boston: Beacon Press, 1966). See *Rediscovering Fuller: Essays on Implicit Law and Institutional Design,* ed. Willem Witteveen and Wibren van der Burg (Amsterdam University Press, 1999); Albert W. Alschuler, *Law without Values: The Life, Work, and Legacy of Justice Holmes* (Chicago: University of Chicago Press, 2000), 150–58. For contemporary wrestling with the presuppositions of law, see generally Steven D. Smith, *Law's Quandary* (Cambridge, MA: Harvard University Press, 2004); Patrick McKinley Brennan, "Realizing the Rule of Law in the Human Subject," *Boston College Law Review,* vol. 43, no. 2 (March 2002), 227–349; Alschuler, *Law without Values;* James Boyd White, *Acts of Hope: Creating Authority in Literature, Law, and Politics* (Chicago: University of Chicago Press, 1994).

6. Norman Maclean, *Young Men and Fire* (Chicago: University of Chicago Press, 1992).

7. Changeux and Connes, *Conversations,* 42. See also Rotman, *Ad Infinitum,* 4–5, 157–58.

8. Michael Polanyi, *The Tacit Dimension* (Garden City, NY: Doubleday, 1966), 3–4.

9. Karl Marx, *Economic and Philosophical Manuscripts,* trans. T. B. Bottomore, in Fromm, *Marx's Concept of Man,* 168. Quoted, in another translation, in George Steiner, *In Bluebeard's Castle: Some Notes towards the Redefinition of Culture* (New Haven: Yale University Press, 1971), 43.

10. Jean-Pierre Changeux, "Drug Use and Abuse," *Daedalus,* vol. 127, no. 2 (Spring 1998), 162; *Neuronal Man: The Biology of Mind,* trans. Laurence Garey (New York: Pantheon Books, 1985), xiv.

11. See Searle, *Rediscovery,* xii, 86–87, *Construction,* xi, 6, 7, and *supra* chapter 3.

Chapter 9.   THE CLAIM OF THE CHILD

1. José Ortega y Gasset, *Toward a Philosophy of History,* trans. Helene Weyl (New York: W. W. Norton, 1941), 14.

2. *The Letters of William Blake with Related Documents,* 3d ed., ed. Geoffrey Keynes (Oxford: Clarendon Press, 1980), 43–46; *The Portable Blake,* ed. with introduction by Alfred Kazin (New York: Penguin, 1976), 210.

3. Jane Kenyon, "Who," in *Otherwise: New and Selected Poems* (St. Paul, MN: Graywolf Press, 1996), 114; William Bolcom, *Briefly It Enters: A Cycle of Songs from the Poems of Jane Kenyon, for Voice and Piano* (Milwaukee: E. B. Marks Music/Bolcom Music, 1997).

4. See, e.g., Allen M. Hornblum, *Acres of Skin: Human Experiments at Holmesburg Prison* (New York: Routledge, 1998); Jon M. Harkness, "Nuremberg and the Issue of Wartime Experiments on U.S. Prisoners," *Journal of the American Medical Association,* vol. 276, no. 20, November 27, 1996, 1672–75. Research funded by the federal Department of Health and Human Services is now guided by regulations, 45 C.F.R. § 46.301 *et seq.,* "Additional Protections Pertaining to Biomedical and Behavioral Research Involving Prisoners as Subjects." Cf. *Kaimowitz v. Michigan Department of Mental Health,* 42 *U.S.L.W.* 2063 (Mich. Cir. Ct. 1973), on the involuntarily committed.

5. See, e.g., Barbara Wooton, *Social Science and Social Pathology* (London: George Allen & Unwin, 1959), 227–67, chapter 8, "Mental Disorder and the Problem of Moral and Criminal Responsibility"; Robert A. Burt, *Taking Care of Strangers: The Rule of Law in Doctor-Patient Relations* (New York: The Free Press, 1979).

6. See, e.g., Victor Klemperer, *I Will Bear Witness: A Diary of the Nazi Years,* vol. 1, 1933–1941, vol. 2, 1941–1945, trans. Martin Chalmers (New York: Random House, 1998, 2000). For an example of debate, compare Daniel Jonah Goldhagen, *Hitler's Willing Executioners: Ordinary Germans and the Holocaust* (New York: Vintage, 1997) with Norman G. Finkelstein and Ruth Bettina Birn, *A Nation on Trial: The Goldhagen Thesis and Historical Truth* (New York: Henry Holt, 1998).

7. "French Children of the Holocaust: A Memorial Exhibition," *New York Times,* February 7, 1997. See also Günther Schwarberg, *The Murders at Bullenhuser Damm: The SS Doctor and the Children* (Bloomington: Indiana University Press, 1984). The reference in "French Children" is to Georges-André Kohn, "taken to the Neuengamme Camp, where he was used in medical experiments and injected with tuberculin bacilli. He was hanged the day before the camp's liberation, in the basement of the Bullenhuser Damm, a school that housed the inhumane human laboratory in Hamburg."

Chapter 10. **THE CLAIM OF THE SPARROW**

1. Alan Lightman and Roberta Brawer, *Origins: The Lives and Worlds of Modern Cosmologists* (Cambridge, MA: Harvard University Press, 1990), 377.

2. Harris, *Factories,* 51; Hal Gold, *Unit 731 Testimony* (Boston and Tokyo: Charles E. Tuttle Co., 1996), 41–42.

3. *New York Times,* March 17, 1995.

4. Ibid.; Harris, *Factories,* 69–70.

5. *New York Times,* March 17, 1995, reporting on 1995 exhibitions about human experimentation in Manchuria. See also Peter Williams and David Wallace, *Unit 731: The Japanese Army's Secret of Secrets* (London: Hodder & Stoughton, 1989), 289.

6. Harris, *Factories,* 109. See also Ralph Blumenthal with Judith Miller, "Japan Rebuffs Requests for Information about Its Germ-Warfare Atrocities," *New York Times,* March 4, 1999; Doug Struck, "Tokyo Court Confirms Japan Used Germ Warfare in China," *Washington Post,* August 28, 2002; Jonathan Watts, "Report," *The Christian Science Monitor,* August 28, 2002.

7. See chapter 6, *supra*; Wade, "Doctors Question Use"; Sun, "EPA Bars Use."

8. David Berreby, "Twists and Turns in Chimp AIDS Research," *New York Times,* February 4, 1997. See also Lawrence K. Altman, "Estrogen Offers Hope Against H.I.V.," *New York Times,* February 1, 2000.

9. Harris, *Factories,* 63.

10. David Berreby, "Unneeded Lab Chimps Face Hazy Future," *New York Times,* February 4, 1997. On sanctuary rather than euthanasia for chimpanzees, see Senate Report No. 106–494, 106th Cong., 2d Sess. (2000), on the Chimpanzee Health Improvement, Maintenance and Protection Act.

11. Berreby, "Unneeded Lab Chimps."

12. Harris, *Factories,* 62, quoting Dong, "Kwantung Army Number 731."

13. *Germany:* Article 20a, in Axel Tschentscher, *The Basic Law (Grundgesetz)* (Würzburg: Jurisprudentia, 2002), 27: "The state, also in its responsibility for future generations, protects the natural foundations of life and the animals in the framework of the constitutional order, by legislation and, according to law and justice, by executive and judiciary." The words "and the animals" were added May 17, 2002, by the 50th Amendment to the Basic Law. See explanatory statement in *Deutscher Bundestag, 14. Wahlperiode, Drucksache 14/8360, 26.02.2002:* "The establishment of a state aim of animal protection takes into account the requirement of morally responsible dealings of humans with animals. The ability to suffer and to feel, especially of more highly developed animals, requires an ethical minimum of human conduct. From that follows the duty to regard animals as fellow beings and to spare them preventable suffering" (trans. B. Tice). *India:* Article 51A(g), in Albert P. Blaustein and Gisbert H. Flanz, eds., *Constitutions of the Countries of the World* (Dobbs Ferry, NY: Oceana Publications, 1994), 81: "It shall be the duty of every citizen of India . . . to have compassion for living creatures." *Florida:* Article X, § 21: "Inhumane treatment of animals is a concern of Florida citizens. To prevent cruelty to certain animals . . . the people of the State of Florida hereby limit. . . ." Amendment adopted Nov. 5, 2002, West's Florida Statutes Annotated, vol. 26A, 2003 Cumulative Annual Pocket Part, 67. *Animal Welfare Act of 1966:* 7 U.S.C. § 2131 *et seq.,* as amended 1970, 1976, 1985, 1990, 2002. For primary legal development in light of this and other federal legislation, see, e.g., *Animal Legal Defense Fund, Inc., et al. v. Glickman,* 154 Fed. 3d 426, 431–38, 444–45 (D.C. Cir. 1998) (en banc) (injury to an individual's interest in the quality of animal life, as distinguished from environmental or ecological interest in the number of animals in existence, held a constitutionally cognizable injury giving rise to an Article III "case or controversy" under the United States Constitution). *Cruelty as Crime:* see, e.g., California Penal Code §§ 597, 599b (West's Annotated California Codes, vol. 49 [1999] with 2002 Cumulative Pocket Part). Cruelty to animals is a felony in the majority of the states of the United States, and may now be statutorily categorized also as a "behavior disorder" (see, e.g., id § 597g [enacted 1998]). *European Union:* Treaty of Amsterdam, October 2, 1997, entered into force May 1, 1999, Protocol on Protection and Welfare of

Animals, "to ensure improved protection and respect for the welfare of animals as sentient beings."

14. E.g., Charles Hartshorne, *Born to Sing: An Interpretation and World Survey of Birdsong* (Bloomington: Indiana University Press, 1973), chapter 12, "Some Philosophical Topics Not Discussed," "Some Conclusions and Unsolved Problems," 226–29; Donald R. Griffin, *Animal Minds* (Chicago: University of Chicago Press, 1992); Alexander F. Skutch, *The Minds of Birds* (College Station: Texas A & M University Press, 1996). Examples of steps taken in the United States toward legal contemplation of an animal as an individual, with an individual life that is not a fungible or replaceable phenomenon, include the Chimpanzee Health Improvement, Maintenance and Protection Act of 2000. The act rejects "euthanasia" of chimpanzees bred in captivity for experiments but no longer needed, and provides for lifetime support of these "surplus chimpanzees" in what is designated as a "sanctuary system." The legislative history notes that the majority report on the matter from the National Research Council "cites the close similarities between chimpanzees and humans." Senate Report No. 106–494. The act itself requires that "none of the chimpanzees may be subjected to euthanasia, except as in the best interests of the chimpanzee involved . . . that the chimpanzees may not be discharged from the system . . . [and] that the Secretary [of the Department of Health and Human Services] may, in the discretion of the Secretary, accept into the system chimpanzees that are not surplus chimpanzees." §§ 481C (d)(2)(I), (J), and (K), Public Law #106–551, December 20, 2000, 42 U.S.C. 287a-3a, 2002 Supplementary Pamphlet.

It may be noted that development in the treatment of animals does not turn on a question of awarding rights. Whether or not a right is spoken of in a case focused on a human being, the legal "merits" of a case concern *public* values if the merits are reached and argued after the jurisdictional stage of the case is concluded. (On this, the reader may find helpful some chapters of my own in *Legal Identity* [New Haven: Yale University Press, 1978], "Private Property and Public Law," and "The Possible Unity of Public and Private Law," 13–33, 179–81). The question currently is principally a question not of rights but of "standing" on the part of those who seek to reach the substantive merits of a challenge to the legality of what is done to an animal—to reach that stage, to have public values argued, and then, if the merits are successfully argued, to enter the remedial or enforcement stage of the case. The degree and scope of recognition of individuality in animals will be pertinent to developments in standing as well as to further legislative, administrative, and other public consideration of what should be done to them.

15. Vicki Hearne, *Adam's Task*; J. M. Coetzee, *The Lives of Animals* (Princeton: Princeton University Press, 1999); Barbara Smuts, "Reflections," in J. M. Coetzee, *The Lives of Animals*, 107–20; Barbara Smuts, "Encounters with Animal Minds," *Journal of Consciousness Studies*, vol. 8, nos. 5–7 (2001), 293–309.

16. "The life within the animal/will give them strength in turn." Eckhart paired animal and child: "If I were alone in a desert/And feeling afraid,/I would want a child to be with me./For then my fear would disappear/And I would be made strong./This is what life in itself can do/because it is so noble, so full of pleasure/And so powerful./But if I could not have a child with me/I would like to have at least a living animal/at my side to comfort me." See Jefferson Powell's reference to his dog Psyche, and to this from Eckhart, in *The Moral Tradition of American Constitutionalism* (Durham: Duke University Press, 1993), ix.

17. The infliction of pain or death on an individual to acquire general knowledge may save the lives of many others in the future. It was this, relative numbers, that was extensively and even eloquently argued at Nuremberg by scientists and doctors to whom the defense of superior orders had scant application. Their defense of their freezing experimental subjects as if in a cold sea and depriving them of oxygen as if falling from a plane was that many more lives were saved by the general knowledge acquired, in Germany and later in America and around the world, than were lost in the experiments. At Nuremberg that was rejected as a defense, and not just in its application to the cases presented there. *Nuernberg Military Tribunals*: "The Medical Case," vol. 1, 114, 124–26, 145–47, 176–77, 200–206, 252, 260, 263, 970–74; vol. 2, 5–6, 10–12, 42–44, 56–77, 181–84.

Nuremberg lies behind the repeated declarations of the World Medical Association in the late twentieth century: "In research on man, the interest of science and society should never take precedence over considerations related to the well-being of the subject." Article III(4), Declarations of Helsinki II(1975), III(1983), IV(1989), V(1996), *Dictionary of Medical Ethics*, A. S. Duncan et al., eds. (London: Darton, Longman & Todd, new rev. ed. 1981), 132–35; III(1983), Dieter Giesen, *International Medical Malpractice Law* (Tübingen: J. C. B. Mohr, 1988), 731–33; IV(1989), 5 *Encyclopedia of Bioethics*, Warren Thomas Reich, ed. (New York: Macmillan, rev. ed. 1995), 2765–67; V(1996), 277 *Journal of the American Medical Association* (March 19, 1997), 925–26. See also the European Convention on Human Rights and Biomedicine, Oviedo, April 4, 1997, European Treaty Series 164, Chapter 1, Article 2: "Primacy of the Human Being: The interests and welfare of the human being shall prevail over the sole interest of society or science." For discussion of the constitutional and common law context in the United States, see generally *Grimes v. Kennedy Krieger Institute, Inc.*, 782 A.2d 807 (Md. 2001) (risky non-therapeutic research on children); *T. D. et al. v. New York State Office of Mental Health*, 626 N.Y.S.2d 1015 (Sup. 1995), 650 N.Y.S.2d 173 (A.D. 1 Dept. 1996), 690 N.E.2d 1259 (N.Y. 1997) (risky non-therapeutic research on the mentally ill).

With regard to severe pain or suffering of an individual as torture, and the question of justification by the number of others benefitted by it, see J. Herman Burgers and Hans Danelius, *The United Nations Convention against Torture: A Handbook on the Convention against Torture and Other Cruel, Inhuman or Degrading Treatment or Punishment* (Dordrecht: Martinus Nijhoff, 1988), 114, 118–19, 123: "Article 1 [of the Convention] does not expressly refer to medical or scientific experiments being carried out on a prisoner against his will and without any therapeutic purpose. This does not exclude, however, that subjecting a person to such experiments could in some cases amount to torture. . . . [I]t may be recalled that Article 7 of the International Convenant on Civil and Political Rights does mention medical or scientific experimentation as a characteristic example of acts violating the prohibition of torture. . . . *Paragraph 2 of Article 2* [of the Convention against Torture] makes it clear that the prohibition of torture is absolute and without exception." Paragraph 2, Article 2: "No exceptional circumstances whatsoever, whether a state of war or a threat of war, internal political instability or other public emergency, may be invoked as a justification of torture."

18. See Stephen Breyer, *Breaking the Vicious Circle: Toward Effective Risk Regulation* (Cambridge, MA: Harvard University Press, 1993).

Further Reading

Alexander, Richard D. *Darwinism and Human Affairs*. Seattle: University of Washington Press, 1982.

Aly, Götz; Chroust, Peter; and Pross, Christian. *Cleansing the Fatherland: Nazi Medicine and Racial Hygiene*. Belinda Cooper, trans. Baltimore: Johns Hopkins University Press, 1994.

Annas, George J., and Grodin, Michael A., eds. *The Nazi Doctors and the Nuremberg Code: Human Rights in Human Experimentation*. New York: Oxford University Press, 1992.

Appleyard, Bryan. *Brave New Worlds: Staying Human in the Genetic Future*. New York: Viking, 1998.

Arnheim, Rudolf. *Parables of Sun Light: Observations on Psychology, the Arts, and the Rest*. Berkeley: University of California Press, 1989.

Barkow, Jerome H.; Cosmides, Leda; and Tooby, John, eds. *The Adapted Mind: Evolutionary Psychology and the Generation of Culture*. New York: Oxford University Press, 1992.

Barrett, William. *Death of the Soul: From Descartes to the Computer*. New York: Anchor Press, 1986.

Barrow, John D. *Theories of Everything: The Quest for Ultimate Explanation*. Oxford: Clarendon Press, 1991.

Barzun, Jacques. *Darwin, Marx, Wagner: Critique of a Heritage*. 2d ed. with a new preface. Chicago: University of Chicago Press, 1981.

———. *A Stroll with William James*. New York: Harper & Row, 1983.

Bateson, Gregory. *Steps to an Ecology of Mind*. New York: Ballantine Books, 1972.

Bauman, Zygmunt. *Modernity and the Holocaust*. Ithaca, NY: Cornell University Press, 1989.

Baumgartner, Peter, and Payr, Sabine, eds. *Speaking Minds: Interviews with Twenty Eminent Cognitive Scientists*. Princeton: Princeton University Press, 1995.

Becker, A. L. *Beyond Translation: Essays toward a Modern Philology.* Ann Arbor: University of Michigan Press, 1995.

Beecher, Henry K. *Research and the Individual: Human Studies.* Boston: Little, Brown, 1970.

Berlin, Isaiah. *The Hedgehog and the Fox: An Essay on Tolstoy's View of History.* London: Weidenfeld & Nicolson, 1953.

———. *Historical Inevitability.* London: Oxford University Press, 1955.

———. *Concepts and Categories: Philosophical Essays.* Henry Hardy, ed. New York: Viking Press, 1979.

Berry, Wendell. *Life Is a Miracle: An Essay against Modern Superstition.* Washington, DC: Counterpoint, 2000.

Blay, Michel. *Reasoning with the Infinite: From the Closed World to the Mathematical Universe.* M. B. DeBevoise, trans. Chicago: University of Chicago Press, 1998.

Blum, Deborah. *Love at Goon Park: Harry Harlow and the Science of Affection.* New York: Perseus, 2002.

Bonner, John T. *The Evolution of Complexity by Means of Natural Selection.* Princeton: Princeton University Press, 1988.

Brown, Andrew. *The Darwin Wars.* London: Simon & Schuster, 1999.

Burgers, J. Herman, and Danelius, Hans. *The United Nations Convention against Torture: A Handbook on the Convention against Torture and Other Cruel, Inhuman or Degrading Treatment or Punishment.* Dordrecht: Martinus Nijhoff, 1988.

Burt, Robert A. *Taking Care of Strangers: The Rule of Law in Doctor-Patient Relations.* New York: The Free Press, 1979.

Byrd, W. Michael, and Clayton, Linda A. *An American Health Dilemma: Race, Medicine, and Health Care in the United States, 1900–2000.* New York: Routledge, 2002.

Calvin, William H. *How Brains Think: Evolving Intelligence, Then and Now.* New York: Basic Books, 1996.

Canetti, Elias. *Crowds and Power.* Carol Stewart, trans. New York: Farrar, Straus and Giroux, 1984.

Caplan, Arthur L., ed. *When Medicine Went Mad: Bioethics and the Holocaust.* Totawa, NJ: Humana Press, 1992.

Changeux, Jean-Pierre. *Neuronal Man: The Biology of Mind.* Laurence Garey, trans. New York: Pantheon Books, 1985.

Changeux, Jean-Pierre, and Connes, Alain. *Conversations on Mind, Matter, and Mathematics.* M. B. DeBevoise, ed. and trans. Princeton: Princeton University Press, 1995.

Changeux, Jean-Pierre, and Ricoeur, Paul. *What Makes Us Think? A Neu-roscientist and a Philosopher Argue about Ethics, Human Nature, and the Brain*. M. B. DeBevoise, trans. Princeton: Princeton University Press, 2000.

Churchland, Paul M. *The Engine of Reason, the Seat of the Soul: A Philo-sophical Journey into the Brain*. Cambridge, MA: MIT Press, 1995.

Clark, Stephen R. L. *The Moral Status of Animals*. Oxford: Clarendon Press, 1977.

———. *Civil Peace and Sacred Order: Limits and Renewals I*. Oxford: Clar-endon Press, 1989.

———. *Biology and Christian Ethics*. Cambridge: Cambridge University Press, 2000.

Clifford, William K. *The Common Sense of the Exact Sciences*. New York: Alfred A. Knopf, 1946; New York: Dover Publications, Inc., 1955.

Coetzee, J. M. *The Lives of Animals*. Princeton: Princeton University Press, 1999.

Commission on the Life Sciences, University of Michigan. *Challenges and Opportunities in Understanding the Complexity of Living Systems*, 1999.

Crick, Francis. *The Astonishing Hypothesis: The Scientific Search for the Soul*. New York: Charles Scribner's Sons, 1994.

Damasio, Antonio R. *Descartes' Error: Emotion, Reason, and the Human Brain*. New York: Avon Books, 1994.

Davis, John. *Exchange*. Minneapolis: University of Minnesota Press, 1992.

Dear, Peter. *Discipline and Experience: The Mathematical Way in the Sci-entific Revolution*. Chicago: University of Chicago Press, 1995.

de Duve, Christian. *Vital Dust: Life as a Cosmic Imperative*. New York: Basic Books, 1996.

Deichmann, Ute. *Biologists under Hitler*. Thomas Dunlap, trans. Cam-bridge, MA: Harvard University Press, 1996.

Dennett, Daniel C. *Darwin's Dangerous Idea: Evolution and the Meanings of Life*. New York: Simon & Schuster, 1995.

de Waal, Frans. *Good Natured: The Origins of Right and Wrong in Humans and Other Animals*. Cambridge, MA: Harvard University Press, 1996.

Dick, Philip K. *Do Androids Dream of Electric Sheep?* New York: Double-day, 1968; New York: Ballantine Books, 1996.

Dikötter, Frank. *Imperfect Conceptions: Medical Knowledge, Birth Defects, and Eugenics in China*. New York: Columbia University Press, 1998.

Dobbs, Betty Jo Teeter. *The Janus Faces of Genius: The Role of Alchemy in Newton's Thought*. Cambridge: Cambridge University Press, 1991.

Dostoyevsky, Fyodor. *The Brothers Karamazov.* Richard Pevear and Larissa Volokhonsky, trans. New York: Alfred A. Knopf, 1992.

Dyson, Freeman. *Disturbing the Universe.* New York: Harper & Row, 1979.

———. *Infinite in All Directions.* New York: Harper & Row, 1988.

———. *Imagined Worlds.* Cambridge, MA: Harvard University Press, 1997.

Edelman, Gerald M. *Bright Air, Brilliant Fire: On the Matter of the Mind.* New York: Basic Books, 1992.

Endo, Shusaku. *The Sea and Poison.* Michael Gallagher, trans. London: Peter Owen, 1995.

Faden, Ruth R., Committee Chair. *U.S. Advisory Committee on Human Radiation Experiments: Final Report.* Washington, DC: U.S. Government Printing Office, 1995.

Faden, Ruth R., and Beauchamp, Tom L. *A History and Theory of Informed Consent.* New York: Oxford University Press, 1986.

Fried, Charles. *Medical Experimentation: Personal Integrity and Social Policy.* Amsterdam: North-Holland, 1974.

Gell-Mann, Murray. *The Quark and the Jaguar: Adventures in the Simple and the Complex.* New York: W. H. Freeman, 1994.

Goodenough, Ursula. *The Sacred Depths of Nature.* New York: Oxford University Press, 1998.

Gould, Stephen Jay. *Ever Since Darwin: Reflections in Natural History.* New York: W. W. Norton, 1977.

———. *Wonderful Life: The Burgess Shale and the Nature of History.* London: Hutchinson Radius, 1989.

Granit, Ragnar; Pannenberg, Wolfhart; Popper, Sir Karl; Rorty, Richard; Wheeler, John Archibald; Wigner, Eugene. *Mind in Nature.* Richard Q. Elvee, ed. San Francisco: Harper & Row, 1982.

Griffin, Donald R. *The Question of Animal Awareness: Evolutionary Continuity of Mental Experience.* New York: Rockefeller University Press, 1981.

———. *Animal Minds.* Chicago: University of Chicago Press, 1992.

Grodin, Michael A., and Glantz, Leonard H., eds. *Children as Research Subjects: Science, Ethics, and Law.* New York: Oxford University Press, 1994.

Gross, Paul R., and Levitt, Norman. *The Higher Superstition: The Academic Left and Its Quarrels with Science.* Baltimore: John Hopkins University Press, 1994.

Gross, Paul R.; Levitt, Norman; and Lewis, Martin W., eds. *The Flight from Science and Reason.* New York: New York Academy of Sciences, 1996.

Haldane, J. B. S. *Possible Worlds.* London: Chatto and Windus, 1927.

Hardy, G.H. *A Mathematician's Apology*. Foreword by C.P. Snow. Cambridge: Cambridge University Press, 1967.

Harris, Roy. *The Language Machine*. Ithaca, NY: Cornell University Press, 1987.

Harris, Sheldon H. *Factories of Death: Japanese Biological Warfare, 1932–1945, and the American Cover-Up*. London: Routledge, 1994.

Hartshorne, Charles. *Born to Sing: An Interpretation and World Survey of Birdsong*. Bloomington: Indiana University Press, 1973.

Hawking, Stephen W. *A Brief History of Time: From the Big Bang to Black Holes*. Introduction by Carl Sagan. New York: Bantam Books, 1988.

Hawking, Stephen W., and Penrose, Roger. *The Nature of Space and Time*. Princeton: Princeton University Press, 1996.

Hearne, Vicki. *Adam's Task: Calling Animals by Name*. New York: Vintage Books, 1986.

Heller, Eric. *The Disinherited Mind*. Harmondsworth: Penguin, 1961.

Hoffman, Roald. *The Same and Not the Same*. New York: Columbia University Press, 1995.

Holland, John H. *Emergence: From Chaos to Order*. Reading, MA: Addison-Wesley, 1998.

Holton, Gerald. *Science and Anti-Science*. Cambridge, MA: Harvard University Press, 1993.

Hornblum, Allen M. *Acres of Skin: Human Experiments at Holmesburg Prison*. New York: Routledge, 1998.

Humphrey, Nicholas. *A History of the Mind: Evolution and the Birth of Consciousness*. New York: HarperCollins, 1993.

Jaccottet, Philippe. *Landscapes with Absent Figures*. Mark Treharne, trans. Preface by Michael Hamburger. London: Menard Press, 1997.

Jacob, François. *The Logic of Life: A History of Heredity*. Betty S. Spillmann, trans. London: Penguin, 1982.

———. *The Possible and the Actual*. Betty S. Spillmann, trans. London: Penguin, 1982.

Johnson-Laird, Philip N. *The Computer and the Mind: An Introduction to Cognitive Science*. Cambridge, MA: Harvard University Press, 1988.

Jonas, Hans. "Philosophical Reflections on Experimenting with Human Subjects," in *Experimentation with Human Subjects*, Paul A. Freund, ed. New York: George Braziller, 1970.

Jones, James H. *Bad Blood: The Tuskegee Syphilis Experiment*. New York: The Free Press, 1993.

Josipovici, Gabriel. *Touch*. New Haven: Yale University Press, 1996.

Kahn, Jeffrey P.; Mastroianni, Anna C.; Sugarman, Jeremy, eds. *Beyond Consent: Seeking Justice in Research*. New York: Oxford University Press, 1998.

Kane, Gordon. *The Particle Garden: Our Universe as Understood by Particle Physicists*. New York: Addison-Wesley, 1995.

Kass, Leon R. *Toward a More Natural Science: Biology and Human Affairs*. New York: The Free Press, 1985.

Kater, Michael H. *Doctors under Hitler*. Chapel Hill: University of North Carolina Press, 1989.

Kean, Hilda. *Animal Rights: Political and Social Change in Britain since 1800*. London: Reaktion Books, 1998.

Kevles, Daniel J. *In the Name of Eugenics: Genetics and the Uses of Human Heredity*. Cambridge, MA: Harvard University Press, 1995.

Klemperer, Victor. *I Will Bear Witness: A Diary of the Nazi Years*. Vol. 1, 1933–1941. Vol. 2, 1941–1945. Martin Chalmers, trans. New York: Random House, 1998, 2000.

———. *The Language of the Third Reich: A Philologist's Notebook*. Martin Brady, trans. London: Continuum, 2002.

Köhler, Wolfgang. "Man and Nature," in *The Place of Value in a World of Facts*, 370–413. New York: Liveright, 1938.

Lakatos, Imre. *Proofs and Refutations: The Logic of Mathematical Discovery*. John Worral and Elie Zahar, eds. Cambridge: Cambridge University Press, 1976.

Lash, Nicolas. *Voices of Authority*. London: Sheed and Ward, 1976.

Lederer, Susan E. *Subjected to Science: Human Experimentation in America before the Second World War*. Baltimore: Johns Hopkins University Press, 1995.

Levine, George. *Darwin and the Novelists: Patterns of Science in Victorian Fiction*. Cambridge, MA: Harvard University Press, 1988; Chicago: University of Chicago Press, 1992.

———. *Dying to Know: Scientific Epistemology and Narrative in Victorian England*. Chicago: University of Chicago Press, 2002.

Lewis, C. S. *Miracles*. New York: Simon & Schuster, 1996.

Lifton, Robert Jay. *The Nazi Doctors: Medical Killing and the Psychology of Genocide*. New York: Basic Books, 1986.

Lightman, Alan, and Brawer, Roberta. *Origins: The Lives and Worlds of Modern Cosmologists*. Cambridge, MA: Harvard University Press, 1990.

Linzey, Andrew. *Animal Theology*. Urbana: University of Illinois Press, 1995.

MacIntyre, Alasdair. *Dependent Rational Animals: Why Human Beings Need the Virtues*. Chicago: Open Court Publishing, 2001.

Macquarrie, John. *God-Talk: An Examination of the Language and Logic of Theology.* London: SCM Press, 1967.

Maitland, Sara. *A Big Enough God: A Feminist's Search for a Joyful Theology.* New York: Riverhead Books, 1996.

McGinn, Colin. *The Character of Mind.* Oxford: Oxford University Press, 1982.

———. *The Mysterious Flame: Conscious Minds in a Material World.* New York: Basic Books, 1999.

Midgley, Mary. *Evolution as a Religion: Strange Hopes and Stranger Fears.* London: Methuen, 1985.

———. *Science and Poetry.* London: Routledge, 2001.

Monod, Jacques. *Chance and Necessity: An Essay on the Natural Philosophy of Modern Biology.* Austryn Wainhouse, trans. New York: Alfred A. Knopf, 1971.

Moravec, Ivan. *Mind Children: The Future of Robot and Human Intelligence.* Cambridge, MA: Harvard University Press, 1988.

Moreno, Jonathan D. *Undue Risk: Secret State Experiments on Humans.* New York: W. H. Freeman, 1999.

Morris, Simon Conway. *Life's Solution: Inevitable Humans in a Lonely Universe.* Cambridge: Cambridge University Press, 2003.

Murdock, Iris. *The Sovereignty of Good.* London: Routledge, 1970.

National Academy of Sciences. *Teaching about Evolution and the Nature of Science.* Washington, DC: National Academy Press, 1998.

National Research Council Committee on Long-Term Care of Chimpanzees. *Chimpanzees in Research: Strategies for Their Ethical Care, Management, and Use.* Washington, DC: National Academy Press, 1997.

New York State Commissioner of Health Advisory Work Group on Human Subject Research Involving the Protected Classes. *Recommendations on the Oversight of Human Subject Research Involving the Protected Classes,* 1998.

Noonan, John T., Jr. "The Alliance of Law and History," in *Persons and Masks of the Law,* 152–67. New York: Farrar, Straus and Giroux, 1976.

———. "Posner's Problematics." *Harvard Law Review* 111, no. 7 (May 1998): 1768–75.

Ortega y Gasset, José. *Toward a Philosophy of History.* New York: W. W. Norton, 1941.

Osserman, Robert. *Poetry of the Universe: A Mathematical Exploration of the Cosmos.* New York: Doubleday, 1995.

Penrose, Roger. *The Emperor's New Mind: Concerning Computers, Minds, and the Laws of Physics.* Oxford: Oxford University Press, 1989.

————. *Shadows of the Mind: A Search for the Missing Science of Consciousness.* Oxford: Oxford University Press, 1994.

Pepperberg, Irene M. *The Alex Studies: Cognitive and Communicative Abilities of Grey Parrots.* Cambridge, MA: Harvard University Press, 1999.

Pernick, Martin S. *The Black Stork: Eugenics and the Death of "Defective" Babies in American Medicine and Motion Pictures since 1915.* New York: Oxford University Press, 1996.

Pippard, Brian. "Master-minding the Universe" (reviewing Paul Davies, *God and the New Physics*). *Times Literary Supplement,* July 29, 1983, 795–96.

Polanyi, Michael. *The Tacit Dimension.* Garden City, NY: Doubleday, 1966.

————. *Personal Knowledge: Towards a Post-Critical Philosophy.* Chicago: University of Chicago Press, 1958; New York: Atheneum, 1990.

Polkinghorne, John. *The Faith of a Physicist.* Princeton: Princeton University Press, 1994.

Pollack, Robert. *The Faith of Biology & the Biology of Faith: Order, Meaning, and Free Will in Modern Medical Science.* New York: Columbia University Press, 2000.

Powell, H. Jefferson. *A Community Built on Words: The Constitution in History and Politics.* Chicago: University of Chicago Press, 2002.

Priest, Graham. *Beyond the Limits of Thought.* Cambridge: Cambridge University Press, 1995.

Proctor, Robert. *Racial Hygiene.* Cambridge, MA: Harvard University Press, 1988.

Pross, Christian, and Aly, Götz. *The Value of the Human Being: Medicine in Germany, 1918–1945.* Marc Iwand, trans. Berlin: Ärztekammer Berlin, 1991.

Regan, Tom, ed. *Animal Sacrifices.* Philadelphia: Temple University Press, 1986.

Reichenbach, Hans. *The Rise of Scientific Philosophy.* Berkeley: University of California Press, 1958.

Richards, Robert J. *Darwin and the Emergence of Evolutionary Theories of Mind and Behavior.* Chicago: University of Chicago Press, 1987.

Rothman, David J. *Strangers at the Bedside: A History of How Law and Bioethics Transformed Medical Decision Making.* New York: Basic Books, 1991.

Rotman, Brian. *Ad Infinitum: The Ghost in Turing's Machine.* Stanford: Stanford University Press, 1993.

Sacks, Oliver. *The Man Who Mistook His Wife for a Hat and Other Clinical Tales.* New York: HarperCollins, 1987.

————. *An Anthropologist on Mars.* New York: Vintage Books, 1995.

————. *Awakenings*. New York: Vintage Books, 1999.

Schwarberg, Günther. *The Murders at Bullenhuser Damm: The SS Doctor and the Children*. Erna Baber Rosenfeld, trans. Bloomington: Indiana University Press, 1984.

Scully, Matthew. *Dominion: The Power of Man, the Suffering of Animals, and the Call to Mercy*. New York: St. Martin's Press, 2002.

Searle, John R. *The Rediscovery of the Mind*. Cambridge, MA: MIT Press, 1992.

————. *The Construction of Social Reality*. New York: The Free Press, 1995.

Sherrard, Philip. *The Eclipse of Man and Nature: An Enquiry into the Origins and Consequences of Modern Science*. West Stockbridge, MA: Lindesfarne Press, 1987.

Silver, Lee M. *Remaking Eden: Cloning and beyond in a Brave New World*. New York: Avon Books, 1997.

Simon, Herbert A. *The Sciences of the Artificial*. 2d ed. Cambridge, MA: MIT Press, 1981.

Skutch, Alexander F. *The Minds of Birds*. College Station: Texas A & M University Press, 1996.

Smith, Steven D. *Foreordained Failure*. New York: Oxford University Press, 1995.

————. *The Constitution and the Pride of Reason*. New York: Oxford University Press, 1998.

————. *Law's Quandary*. Cambridge, MA: Harvard University Press, 2004.

Smuts, Barbara. "Encounters with Animal Minds." *Journal of Consciousness Studies* 8, no. 5–7 (2001): 293–309.

Steiner, George. *In Bluebeard's Castle: Some Notes towards the Redefinition of Culture*. New Haven: Yale University Press, 1971.

————. *Real Presences*. Chicago: University of Chicago Press, 1989.

Tallis, Raymond. *The Explicit Animal: A Defence of Human Consciousness*. London: Macmillan, 1991.

————. *Psycho-Electronics*. London: Ferrington, 1994.

————. *Newton's Sleep: The Two Cultures and the Two Kingdoms*. London: Macmillan, 1995.

Taylor, Charles. *Sources of the Self: The Making of the Modern Identity*. Cambridge, MA: Harvard University Press, 1989.

————. *A Catholic Modernity?* New York: Oxford University Press, 1999.

Teichman, Jenny. *The Mind and the Soul: An Introduction to the Philosophy of Mind*. London: Routledge & Kegan Paul, 1974.

Thomas, Lewis. *The Lives of a Cell: Notes of a Biology Watcher*. New York: Bantam Books, 1974.

————. *The Medusa and the Snail: More Notes of a Biology Watcher.* New York: Bantam Books, 1980.

————. *Late Night Thoughts on Listening to Mahler's Ninth Symphony.* New York: Viking, 1983.

————. *Et Cetera, Et Cetera: Notes of a Word-Watcher.* New York: Penguin, 1990.

————. *The Fragile Species.* New York: Macmillan, 1992.

Thompson, D'Arcy. *On Growth and Form.* Abridged ed. Introduction by J. T. Bonner. Cambridge: Cambridge University Press, 1975.

Toulmin, Stephen. *The Return to Cosmology: Postmodern Science and the Theology of Nature.* Berkeley: University of California Press, 1982.

Turner, James C. *Reckoning with the Beast: Animals, Pain, and Humanity in the Victorian Mind.* Baltimore: Johns Hopkins University Press, 1980.

Veyne, Paul. *Did the Greeks Believe in Their Myths?: An Essay on the Constitutive Imagination.* Paula Wissing, trans. Chicago: University of Chicago Press, 1988.

Vickers, Geoffrey. *The Art of Judgment: A Study of Policy Making.* London: Chapman & Hall, 1965.

Vining, Joseph. *The Authoritative and the Authoritarian.* Chicago: University of Chicago Press, 1986.

————. *From Newton's Sleep.* Princeton: Princeton University Press, 1995.

————. "Fuller and Language," in *Rediscovering Fuller: Essays on Implicit Law and Institutional Design.* Willem Witteveen and Wibren van der Burg, eds. Amsterdam: Amsterdam University Press, 1999.

Walker, Stephen. *Animal Thought.* London: Routledge, 1983.

Weinberg, Steven. *Dreams of a Final Theory.* New York: Pantheon Books, 1992.

————. *The First Three Minutes: A Modern View of the Origin of the Universe.* Updated ed. New York: Basic Books, 1993.

Weinreb, Lloyd L. *Natural Law and Justice.* Cambridge, MA: Harvard University Press, 1987.

Weizenbaum, Joseph. *Computer Power and Human Reason: From Judgment to Calculation.* New York: W. H. Freeman, 1976.

Westfall, Richard S. *The Life of Isaac Newton.* Cambridge: Cambridge University Press, 1993.

White, James Boyd. *Justice as Translation: An Essay in Cultural and Legal Criticism.* Chicago: University of Chicago Press, 1990.

————. *Acts of Hope: Creating Authority in Literature, Law, and Politics.* Chicago: University of Chicago Press, 1994.

————. *From Expectation to Experience: Essays on Law and Legal Education.* Ann Arbor: University of Michigan Press, 2000.

————. *The Edge of Meaning.* Chicago: University of Chicago Press, 2001.

Wilson, Edward O. *On Human Nature.* Cambridge, MA: Harvard University Press, 1978.

————. *Consilience: The Unity of Knowledge.* New York: Alfred A. Knopf, 1998.

Wolf, Susan. *Freedom within Reason.* New York: Oxford University Press, 1990.

Wolpert, Lewis. "Science and Anti-Science." *Journal of the Royal College of Physicians of London* 21, no. 2 (1987): 159–65.

Index

acknowledgment of person: in general, 21, 91, 124, 126; human language and, 160–62n2; in scientific thought, 65, 85–91, 93, 95

action: as perception, 79, 130; and reading of belief, 2, 12, 49, 57, 78, 83, 99, 125, 136, 139, 140; and responsibility, 87–88; as understanding another, 117–18, 121–22

adolescence, pattern of, 56, 76–77

aesthetics: and the brain, 43; Darwin and, 27; relativism in, 45

agency, and authority, 104

alikeness: and the future, 32–33; individual judgment of, 106; insanity and, 127–28; and knowledge of death, 133; and the line, 82, 98, 123–27, 131; and newness, 126; as not alone, 126; terms of, 143; two directions of, 78, 126, 130, 149–50

aloneness, 15; alikeness and, 106, 126; and authority, 106, 126; individuality and, 117; manipulation and, 89; and purpose, 133–34; and search for life beyond earth, 144

altruism, 133; and cosmology, 103; and evolution, 34; experiments on, 56; sense of, 97, 143, 147, 149

animals: and consciousness, 140, 169n14; cruelty toward, as crime, 139, 168n13; differences among, 141; experimentation on, 2, 5, 6, 12, 46, 47, 56, 114, 138, 140; faithfulness to, 120; human beings as, 7, 10, 26, 40, 48, 82, 124, 129, 164n2; legal protection of, 139, 168n13; legal standing to speak for, 168n13, 169n14; and the line, 124, 136, 140; mourning among, 145; recognition of individuality by, 140; recognition of individuality of, 150, 159n9, 169n14; as sentient beings, 140, 168–69n13; twentieth-century study of, 139–40, 169n14

Antigone (Sophocles), 106

antiscience, 2, 12, 50, 63, 85, 91, 135; close reading and, 133; dependence of, on sense of science, 59, 69, 122; Jacques Monod on, 25, 50; possibility of, 2, 12, 72, 85, 91; sources of, 26, 41; Lewis Thomas on, 24

anti-Semitism: and dehumanization, 26, 75–76; explaining challenge to itself, 42; tone of, 45

apology: of lawyer, 17; of mathematician, 17, 95

JOSEPH VINING

is Hutchins Professor of Law at the University of Michigan.

THE SONG SPARROW AND THE CHILD

was composed in 10.9/13.2 Fairfield
on a G4 Macintosh using QuarkXPress 4.1
at Four Star Books;
printed by sheet-fed offset
on 55# EcoBook 100 Antique stock
(100% post-consumer recycled, processed chlorine free),
smyth sewn bound over binder's boards
in Rainbow 3 cloth,
and wrapped with dust jackets printed in two colors
on 80# enamel stock finished with film lamination
by Thomson-Shore, Inc.;
designed by Wendy McMillen;
and published by the
University of Notre Dame Press
Notre Dame, Indiana 46556

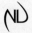